Lyme Disease

A Johns Hopkins Press Health Book

Lyme Disease

The Cause, the Cure, the Controversy

ALAN G. BARBOUR, M.D.

The Johns Hopkins University Press
Baltimore and London

Note to the reader: This book is not meant to substitute for medical care of people with Lyme disease, and treatment should not be based solely on its contents. Instead, treatment must be developed in a dialogue between the individual and his or her physician. This book has been written to help with that dialogue.

The cases of Lyme disease and chronic fatigue syndrome discussed in this book are not those of actual individuals, and any resemblance to actual individuals is purely coincidental. The case histories are composites from true case histories and are meant to illustrate certain aspects of Lyme disease.

© 1996 The Johns Hopkins University Press
All rights reserved. Published 1996
Printed in the United States of America on acid-free paper

05 04 03 02 01 00 99 98 97 96   5 4 3 2 1

The Johns Hopkins University Press
2715 North Charles Street
Baltimore, Maryland 21218-4319
The Johns Hopkins Press Ltd., London

Library of Congress Cataloging-in-Publication Data will be found at the end of this book.

A catalog record for this book is available from the British Library.

ISBN 0-8018-5224-2
ISBN 0-8018-5245-5 (pbk.)

Contents

Illustrations

Preface and Acknowledgments

I had three principal motivations in undertaking this project. The first and most specific was a desire to try to set the record straight. The public as well as health professionals are often confused by the conflicting opinions expressed about various aspects of Lyme disease, and this misunderstanding contributes to the Lyme disease problem. When a disease is poorly defined, it's inevitable that there will be controversies—about what the illness is and how it should be managed, for example. Under these circumstances, it's not surprising that people become frustrated and seek answers from a variety of sources.

My second reason was more general, and that was to increase people's understanding that the potential for diseases to be acquired from nature is currently underestimated. At the millennium people seem to be more afraid of what other people can do to them— through crime, terrorism, and governmental regulations, for example—than of anything in the natural world. Many people believe that the answer to our problems lies in a return to a more agrarian society—or even to the hunter-gatherer stage of human history. But this nostalgic view overlooks present and potential hazards from contacts with nature. As civilization further extends itself into the wilderness and jungles of the developing world, and as cities encroach farther and farther into the woods and forests in the developed world, people already are coming into direct contact with the microorganisms of those less tame environs. AIDS and Ebola virus infection are two recent examples of what can happen when microorganisms move from wildlife to people. Lyme disease is another example, and the one with which I am now most familiar.

My third reason for writing the book was even broader, and

stemmed from my conviction that most scientists and physicians don't make a sufficient effort to explain to people outside their fields of inquiry—including their own patients and family members—about the processes of scientific research and medical decision making. There are books about various diseases, and there are books about fascinating discoveries in physics or neuroscience. But it seems to me that in these books the complexities and uncertainties of a field are often glossed over in the effort to try to make the subject accessible. I think that people can make good decisions about health matters for themselves or for others only when they are fully informed—when as many cards as possible are face up on the table. Only under these circumstances can people assess the different sides in a technical controversy, and this is especially important when the fields are medicine and disease prevention.

In developing this project, I looked to my own experience as well as the experience of others. I am not an expert in all matters about Lyme disease, and in order to write about those areas that are not in my immediate command, I sought out the advice of experts in those fields. Because there are so many controversies regarding the disease, some people will probably take exception to what I wrote or what I chose not to write. Although I have tried to be comprehensive in this book, inevitably and regrettably I almost certainly have omitted some information, either because the finding was unknown to all at the time of writing—mid-1995—or because I overlooked it.

In some cases I have expressed my own opinion, whether it is the generally accepted opinion or not; but in most cases where there are disputes within the scientific community, I have expressed the opinion that was best supported by the available scientific data. Some unproven theories and ideas are very appealing, but they are difficult to recommend if the only basis for their acceptance at this point is anecdotal. Compelling stories, many of them from patients, should be taken seriously: they may point the direction to new concepts of disease and treatment. But ultimately those holding views that are contrary to what has been shown scientifically must put their own theories to the test. I hope that this book will serve in part to promote the value of testing, clinically, new diagnostic approaches and treatments for Lyme disease.

When I told my medical and research colleagues that I was writing a book on Lyme disease for the general public, most of them expressed surprise that I could find the time in the day to do this, considering all the other demands of academic life. They may be right, and I may have neglected certain aspects of a university career in doing so. (Advancement at research institutions is seldom secured by writing a book for the general public.) If I had produced a technical book for my peers, my motives might have been more comprehensible. But I found the three motives described above to be compelling indeed.

Numerous mentors, colleagues, friends, and students have over the years, through their own research, by their example, or by their dedication, revealed to me much of what I know about the Lyme disease phenomenon and *Borrelia* infections. Those who stand out are Rudolf Ackermann, John Anderson, Eva Åsbrink, Jorge Benach, Sven Bergström, Willy Burgdorfer, Lisa Dever, Paul Duray, Brian Fallon, Mehdi Ferdows, Durland Fish, Claude Garon, Klaus Hansen, Joe Hinnebusch, Timothy Howe, Russell Johnson, Todd Kitten, Edward Korenberg, Robert Lane, Paul Lavoie, Kenneth Leigner, Ben Luft, Lou Magnarelli, Edwin Masters, Leonard Mayer, Polly Murray, Andrew Pachner, Joe Piesman, Blanca Restrepo, Ariadna Sadziene, Steve Schutzer, Tom Schwan, Leonard Sigal, Andrew Spielman, Gerold Stanek, Allen Steere, Gören Stiernstedt, Herbert Stoenner, John Swanson, Karen Vanderhoof-Forschner, Klaus Weber, David Weld, Bettina Wilske, Gary Wormser, and Martina Ziska. My research on spirochetes and Lyme disease has been supported by the National Institutes of Health, the National Science Foundation, the Arthritis Foundation, Connaught Laboratories, Inc., and the Lyme Disease Foundation.

For reading all or parts of the manuscript and for providing helpful suggestions (which I did not always follow) I thank Anita Barbour, George Barbour, Sven Bergström, Roy Campbell, David Dennis, Durland Fish, Steve Hill, William Matuzas, Ed McSweegan, Ann

Meredith, Joe Piesman, Ariadna Sadziene, Jeff Slade, Chuck So-haskey, Gerold Stanek, and Allen Steere. For helping me through the figurative gestation and delivery I thank my editor, Jacqueline Wehmueller, and my copyeditor, Miriam Kleiger. Finally, I could never have started—let alone completed—the book without the encouragement, support, and patience of my wife, Ann, and my sons, Evan and Nathan.

Introduction

Just by virtue of living in the world, human beings are susceptible to disease. Many diseases—for example, influenza and tuberculosis—are spread when bacteria or viruses pass from one person to another. Other diseases are acquired genetically, from one's parents; one of these is cystic fibrosis. Some diseases, such as coronary heart disease and osteoporosis, develop as we age. Others we get from the environment; examples are lead poisoning, and skin cancer due to exposure to the sun. Finally, there are diseases that can be transmitted from animals to humans. Lyme disease is one such disease.

In Lyme disease (sometimes called Lyme borreliosis), ticks transmit the infection from animals to humans. Ticks normally feed on wildlife or domestic animals, but they do sometimes also bite humans and their pets. While the ticks are feeding, pathogenic (disease-producing) microorganisms called spirochetes (pronounced *spiro-keets*) enter the skin. In this case they are spirochetes of *Borrelia burgdorferi* (*B. burgdorferi*, for short), which is the bacterium that causes Lyme disease.

When ticks transmit *B. burgdorferi* to humans, a rash develops where the spirochetes enter the skin. Several days to weeks later, there may be symptoms elsewhere in the body, where the spirochetes have spread. The symptoms are more likely to appear in the joints, the nervous system, and the heart than anywhere else in the body. When the symptoms of Lyme disease appear in these parts of the body, the person may be considerably disabled. It is this potential for disability that, understandably, makes people so afraid of the disease.

Lyme disease is common in parts of North America, Europe, and Asia. Of all the infections that are passed from ticks or insects to humans in the United States, Canada or Europe, Lyme disease is the most common. But the risk of becoming infected is not the same in different parts of the United States. Most cases of Lyme disease have occurred along the northeast coast, in parts of the upper Midwest, and in northern California. Curiously, some regions of the country report many cases of Lyme disease even though few or none of the ticks that carry the disease have been found there.

Looking back, we can see that Lyme disease, in one form or another, was recognized by physicians in Europe beginning in the early twentieth century. In North America, however, it was not until the 1970s that physicians in the United States and Canada began to report that they were seeing patients who had the disease. Whether some people on this continent actually had Lyme disease—not recognized as such—for decades before then is not clear.

Although we know a great deal about Lyme disease—how it is transmitted, what the early symptoms are, and where in this country it is most likely to occur—our understanding of it is still relatively incomplete. There is much that we don't know about how the disease is transmitted by ticks to people and how the spirochetes cause disease. Scientists continue to search for better ways to diagnose the disease and treat people who have it. Misunderstandings about what Lyme disease is and how people get it can lead to confusion—and to misdiagnosis and mistreatment. This may partly explain the puzzling statistic noted above: the fact that many cases of the disease are reported in regions not found to harbor many—or any—of the transmitting ticks.

One of the most confusing aspects of Lyme disease for people is the difficulty in defining precisely what it is. Opinions range from one extreme—the view that Lyme disease is usually a simple infection that is either self-limited or easily treated with a short course of antibiotics—to the other, namely, the belief that the disease often becomes a lifelong affliction that shows little improvement with conventional treatment. Most of those holding the first view believe that Lyme disease, like other well-known infections, such as influenza and gonorrhea, can be confirmed by laboratory tests for either the microorganism itself or the body's immune response to its presence. Many of those holding the other view do not accept negative laboratory tests as evidence that an individual is not ill with Lyme disease.

The controversy over the diagnostic definition of Lyme disease has become so heated that at least one physician's office has been picketed by people who believe that physicians are not taking the threat of the disease seriously enough. Moreover, at least one state legislature has considered a bill that would compel insurance companies to reimburse patients for the lengthy and expensive treatments that are prescribed for the disease by some physicians.

Whatever the merits of these various definitions, there is no disputing that many people have Lyme disease and that many others are worried that they may have it. The symptoms of the disease have been described in newspapers and magazines and on television. Some of these symptoms, such as a localized skin rash followed weeks later by a swollen and painful knee joint, are characteristic of the disease. Other publicized symptoms, such as fatigue, are less specific. That is, they may indicate the presence of a disease, but they do not, on their own, indicate what that disease could be. Because even the most conservative definition of Lyme disease includes such nonspecific symptoms as fatigue and muscle aches, it is not surprising that some people attribute these common symptoms to this infection, especially if the symptoms persist. One reason that people might welcome a diagnosis of Lyme disease rather than other diagnoses is that there is hope for a cure with Lyme disease, since antibiotics usually effectively treat the illness. The outlook is less optimistic for people with other disorders (such as rheumatoid arthritis and multiple sclerosis, for example) that in their early stages might be confused with Lyme disease. And Lyme disease doesn't have the social stigma of some other infectious diseases, such as syphilis, tuberculosis, and AIDS, which might fit these same symptoms. People get Lyme disease as a result of wholesome activities such as hiking in the woods or working in the garden, and so patients aren't embarrassed to ask their physicians whether they might have the disease, or to tell their friends and family that they do.

But what happens when a person with symptoms suggestive of Lyme disease has a blood test whose results indicate that Lyme disease is not causing these symptoms? And what about the person whose symptoms don't entirely disappear with antibiotic therapy? Sometimes an alternative course of therapy is successful in eliminating symptoms, but more often the symptoms persist, or they return after having disappeared for a while. When there is confusion over a diagnosis of Lyme disease, or when the most commonly prescribed treatments do not "cure" the disease, then the patient may be told that he or she does not have it. Some people may even be told that the persistent symptoms are "all in their head."

For a person who had assumed that his or her symptoms were attributable to Lyme disease, and that antibiotics would cure the disease and make the symptoms go away, this is neither welcome information nor an acceptable way to describe their situation. Not surprisingly, the person may become frustrated or angry and may decide to seek the care of a different physician, most likely one who is willing to try another cycle of antibiotics. Some people seek help from alternative medicine practitioners such as acupuncturists and chiropractors.

The encouraging information for people in this situation is that their symptoms probably aren't in their head, and that once the cause of the symptoms is properly diagnosed, treatment to relieve the symptoms is likely to be effective. There are many explanations other than Lyme disease for these common symptoms, and the treatment for the other conditions may be very different from the treatment for Lyme disease. If someone doesn't have Lyme disease, then treating the person for that disease won't work. But if the real cause of the problem is discovered, effective treatment can begin.

There is one thing that all the experts agree on: the best way to control Lyme disease is to prevent it. Essentially, this means stopping the transmission of the disease to people in their yards and recreation areas. Of course, there is disagreement about *how* prevention is to be achieved. For example, the risk of Lyme disease would be much reduced if deer were eliminated from some areas. But any effort to accomplish this would be protested by animal rights activists, hunters, and others. Moreover, reduction or elimination of deer herds requires a community response, and it is often difficult to elicit the cooperation of an entire community.

Another approach to preventing disease puts greater emphasis on the role of the individual, who can take self-protective measures such as using insect repellents and wearing light-colored long-sleeved shirts and long pants when outdoors. Someday a vaccine may protect people from contracting Lyme disease (scientists are working to develop such a vaccine). Applying pesticides to lawns can be effective even for individual homes.

In this book, all of these issues will be explored. Our understanding of Lyme disease—while still limited compared with our knowledge about other infections—is increasing rapidly, and advances in diagnosis and treatment are being made all the time. With what we already know about the disease, you can learn to assess your chances of getting Lyme disease, and you can learn to reduce your risks. If you understand the disease, you will be better prepared to participate in making health care decisions should you become infected. And if you know what other diseases have the same symptoms, you may be better able to accept another diagnosis if Lyme disease turns out not to be causing your illness.

That Lyme disease is controversial there is no doubt; but even where controversy and competing definitions exist, if you know what the different opinions and options are, you have a better chance of making good decisions based on what's best for you. Your physician will play an important role in helping you make these decisions. The purpose of this book is to describe the different opinions and options about the diagnosis and treatment of Lyme disease, in order to help you make decisions about your own health care and prevention of disease.

Lyme Disease

What Is Lyme Disease, and How Do People Get Sick?

- Twelve-year-old Julia and her family lived in a suburb outside of Minneapolis, Minnesota. One summer morning Julia woke with a headache, which lasted through the day. Her mother took her temperature that evening and found it to be a little above normal—100°F. Assuming that Julia had caught the "summer flu" that was going around the neighborhood, her mother gave her an over-the-counter headache medicine. But the next day Julia's headache was worse, she felt tired, and her temperature was still elevated. When Julia came out of the shower, her mother noticed a flat, ring-shaped red rash, five inches in diameter, on the back of her thigh. The edge of the rash was redder than the center. The rash didn't hurt and it didn't itch; in fact, Julia hadn't even noticed it. Julia's mother called her pediatrician's clinic and made an appointment for her daughter that afternoon.

- Werner was a medical student in Vienna, Austria. When he arrived at school one day, a friend told Werner that there was something different about his face. Looking in the mirror, he saw that the right side of his face was drooping. He could not smile or furrow his brow on that side. A week earlier, Werner had started having pain radiating from his shoulder down his right arm, but he had assumed that this was the result of the four sets of competitive tennis he had played. But now the pains were more aggravating. Werner, like many medical students, imagined that he had many of the diseases he had been reading and hearing about. Concerns about multiple sclerosis, stroke, and other equally grave diseases occupied his mind. Later that night, worried that he was seriously ill, he went to the hospital.

- Catherine had lived in Phoenix, Arizona, all her life and played golf on weekends throughout the year. One day in January she was walking down the fairway from the tee when she felt pain in her right knee. When she got home she noticed that her right knee was larger than her left. The joints of her legs and arms had been aching for the last few months, but these aches had come and gone on their own or after treatment with aspirin or ibuprofen. She had been feeling more tired than usual, but this she attributed to the stress of her job. The day after her golf game, when she found that her knee was still swollen and she couldn't walk without limping, Catherine called for an appointment with her physician, who examined her two days later.

- Roy had been drinking more coffee to offset the tiredness he felt during the day, but other than that he hadn't noticed any changes in his health or habits until he began having chills and muscle aches. Even though he didn't feel very well, he decided to go to work anyway, because he had a deadline to meet. He was walking to work from the subway stop in New York City when he fainted onto the sidewalk. Roy had just turned forty-five. Because he had taken up jogging again, he had recently taken a stress test to check his heart's condition. It had indicated that he had no heart problems, so he was surprised when the physicians told him in the emergency room that his heart was beating too slowly and that he needed a pacemaker.

Four people, four different illnesses—yet each of them had Lyme disease. Stories like Julia's are common. Those like Werner's, Catherine's, and Roy's are less common, but they illustrate the more frequent complications of Lyme disease. Although the four illnesses seem to have little in common, in each case—with additional information—a diagnosis of Lyme disease could be made and appropriate therapy begun. But before considering what happened next to these four people, let's go back in time to consider how their infections started.

Lyme Disease Infection and the Immune Response
How Does Lyme Disease Start?

Julia, Werner, Catherine, and Roy were almost certainly bitten by ticks. Each infection started when a tick that had spirochetes in its intestines and saliva glands buried its mouth in the skin to feed on blood (spirochetes are described in more detail in Chapter 3). As the tick remained partially embedded in this way, the spirochetes moved out of the tick into the surrounding skin. This migration usually begins several hours after the tick first attaches itself to the person.

Often people will see the tick while it is feeding and remove it. If they do this during the first day after the tick embeds, there is less chance of infection. In other instances, the tick falls off on its own after its meal. In any case, once the spirochetes have an opportunity to move to the person's skin, the tick's role in these events ends. A residual indication of a tick bite may be a small red bump that lasts for a few days. Some people have allergic reactions to the ticks themselves, in which case the area of redness around the bite may be larger, and it may itch. This is not an infection at all, even though there is redness and swelling. The redness that occurs is similar to a skin hypersensitivity to a cosmetic or to certain metals in jewelry.

Sometimes people do develop an infection at the tick bite, but the infection is not Lyme disease. Such infections can occur after any break or cut in the skin. They are not caused by spirochetes but by other bacteria, such as those that cause strep throat. In these cases the tick cannot be blamed for carrying the disease, because the bacteria usually are on the person's skin when the tick arrives. But by breaking the protective surface of the skin, the tick bite allows the bacteria to infect the person's internal tissues. The infection causes the skin around the tick bite to become red and swollen, and often it becomes very tender. The size of the inflamed area may increase substantially within a matter of hours. The medical term for this type of infection is *cellulitis*. Sometimes cellulitis is confused with early Lyme disease.

But let's assume that Julia, Werner, Catherine, and Roy had neither an allergic reaction to the tick itself nor a cellulitis. If we could look into the skin around where the tick had fed, we would see spirochetes in the spaces between the skin cells. Spirochetes are long, wavy bacteria that have the ability to move and to change direction. They travel as a snake does when it moves over the ground. And like a snake, they can fit into tight spaces, such as those between human

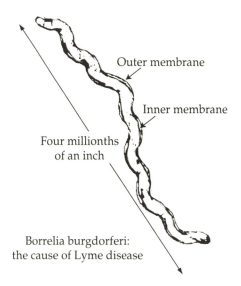

Outer membrane

Inner membrane

Four millionths
of an inch

Borrelia burgdorferi:
the cause of Lyme disease

A *Borrelia burgdorferi* spirochete.

skin cells. Spirochetes require simple sugars, fats, and other substances for energy and growth. Because they cannot make these on their own, they have to get them from the host's surrounding tissues or blood. Most spirochetes are parasites; they take from their host but do not give anything in return. As they divide and multiply within one area of the host's body, they begin to compete among themselves for food resources. Then, in order to survive, they move out from their starting place in order to search for new sources of food. As we will see, however, there is another factor influencing the movement of the spirochetes.

The Early Response to Infection

While the spirochetes are multiplying and feeding, the human who was infected by the tick begins to respond to their presence. This is not a conscious response on the person's part, such as shouting or raising a fist. Instead, the response occurs automatically, with neither the need for nor the possibility of conscious direction. This defense is the *immune response* that occurs when humans are infected with viruses, bacteria, and other microorganisms. An immune response also occurs when a person gets a vaccination, or receives an organ transplant from someone who is not closely related.

If the immune response is successful, the person is said to have *immunity* against the microorganism or cancer. The earliest immune responses to the microorganism's presence tend to be general—that is, their design protects people against a variety of microscopic threats. For example, *lysozyme*, an enzyme in the tear fluid, kills—lyses—certain types of bacteria before they begin to multiply on the surface of the eye. Other natural substances that are "on guard" in the blood neutralize organisms that occasionally enter the bloodstream when we brush our teeth or cut our skin.

If this first line of defense is broached and the infection progresses, humans and other animals respond in another nonspecific way to the invasion. The presence of the bacteria or viruses directly or indirectly stimulates the production of hormonelike substances called *cytokines*, which act as chemical messengers between cells. By releasing a cytokine, a cell can influence the condition or behavior of another cell. Different kinds of cytokines are secreted by different kinds of cells. Cells in the lungs release one type of cytokine, while certain cells in the skin may predominantly make another type.

The cytokine's effect can be local—for example, it can take place between adjacent cells—or it can be long-distance, as, for instance, when cytokines enter the blood and are distributed throughout the body. One cytokine may turn on selected activities in the target cell, while another turns off a different set of activities. Most of the effects of cytokines are on white blood cells (what used to be called corpuscles) and other parts of the immune system. But cytokines can also affect other kinds of cells, such as those in the brain. One cytokine, called IL-1, causes blood vessels to dilate and the body's temperature to rise, and induces sleep. Another cytokine, gamma interferon, which has been developed as a pharmaceutical agent, produced mental depression in several people who were treated with it for cancer.

During the Lyme disease infection the spirochetes seldom if ever become very abundant in the skin or elsewhere in the body (as we will see, this is one reason that Lyme disease is difficult to diagnose). They have an effect on human cells that is out of proportion to their numbers. Scientists have found that proteins on the surface of the spirochete cause human and animal cells to release cytokines in particularly large amounts. Whether spirochetes have anything to gain from stimulating cytokines is not clear. The local result, though, is a red rash like the one Julia had. The skin's redness is due to *inflammation*, a word derived from the Latin word *inflammare*, meaning "to set on fire." There is redness and swelling because the blood vessels dilate and white blood cells move from the blood to the tissues in the area. Cytokines and some hormones bring about inflammation for a purpose, that is, to limit the spread of a foreign invader. The spirochetes, being mobile, may respond to all this activity by moving to tissue that is not yet inflamed. Thus, there are two good reasons for a spirochete's migration: one, to seek out food, and two, to escape the wave of inflammation that it has provoked.

The Skin Rash of Lyme Disease

As the spirochetes move away from the tick bite area, the inflammation response follows them. What started as a small red spot grows, over the next several days to weeks, to become a large patch of red, which is usually circular or oval but may also be triangular. Solitary patches are most commonly found on the trunk or the legs; less often, solitary rashes are discovered on the arms, head, and neck. In dark-skinned individuals the rash may be more difficult to detect because there is less contrast between the rash and the surrounding skin. On any skin, the rash is more likely to be Lyme disease if it is more than two inches (about five centimeters) at its widest.

Because there are fewer spirochetes left behind in the "wake" of the migration, the inner area of the rash sometimes is paler than the edge; the outer border may be bright red. The battle lines have been moved to follow the advance of the spirochetes, and there is now less inflammation in the center. The resulting skin rash was given the name *erythema chronicum migrans* by European physicians at the start of this century. This Latin term means "long-lasting red rash that increases in size." The rash is now more often called simply "erythema migrans," or "EM" for short. By either name, the ring-like rash is typical enough that physicians often can make the diagnosis of Lyme disease solely from the appearance of the rash and the patient's story.

An occasional variation on the expanding-ring pattern is a rash that looks like a target. Rather than one ring, two or three distinct rings surround a paler center. This pattern is also suggestive of Lyme disease, especially if, like the ring rash or large red patch, the target rash is not particularly painful or itchy. A few patients have rashes that are less typical of Lyme disease. Rarely, there may be small blisters in the rash. (A skin rash that is very dry and scaly is not likely to be a sign of Lyme disease.) At least 20 percent of patients with Lyme disease do not remember having seen a rash. A physician who examines a person with an atypical rash or no rash at all is necessarily less confident of the diagnosis.

If untreated, the ringlike rash or patch may grow during the next two to four weeks until it is more than a foot in diameter. More commonly, the rash begins to recede on its own after a certain point. Before antibiotics were used for treatment, physicians observed that the erythema migrans rash disappeared after several days or a few weeks. How could this occur, since the spirochetes are so adept at staying one step ahead of the advancing inflammation? The explanation lies in the fact that the person eventually launches a more formidable defense against the infection. The early response in the skin, like early responses in the lungs or intestines, is not specific for the spirochetes. But the later response is a different matter. It is tailor-made to combat the particular type of microorganism that is invading.

The Specific Response to Infection

The delayed, more specific response to the spirochetes is carried out by *antibodies* and *lymphocytes*. Antibodies are the proteins that often are formed after we experience a new or foreign substance in our bodies. The event that introduces the new substance may be an infection—having one bout of influenza protects us against having another bout with the same virus. It might also be a vaccination; after a tetanus shot, we are protected against developing that disease. Antibody proteins derive their specificity from unique regions in their structures. These fit around a part of the influenza virus or a part of the tetanus poison, as a lock fits around a key. We speak of an antibody "recognizing" this or that substance. An antibody that is effective against a tetanus poison is not effective against the influenza virus, and vice versa.

Antibodies that recognize the Lyme disease spirochete may be present in the host body before the infection occurs, but not in large enough numbers to be effective in curbing the spirochetes' initial spread. It may be several days to weeks before there are sufficient numbers of antibodies to launch an adequate attack against the spirochetes. Because the antibodies circulate throughout the body, they provide a wider field of protection than the nonspecific, local defense provided in the skin during early infection. As soon as antibody levels are high enough in an area, the spirochetes cannot outrun them.

If antibodies are one arm of the specific immune defense, the other arm is the lymphocyte. Lymphocytes are a type of white blood cell. When a white blood cell (WBC) count of the blood is performed, it is generally found that lymphocytes make up the majority or a large minority of the white blood cells in the circulation. Some lymphocytes in the body respond in a specific or restricted way to infectious microorganisms. Indeed, one type of lymphocyte produces antibodies. Other lymphocytes do not form antibodies but either help to produce them or perform much as antibodies do, recognizing and attaching themselves to parts of bacteria or viruses. Like an antibody, a lymphocyte of this type can respond only to that molecule or part of a cell for which it is particularly fitted. The contribution of this type of lymphocyte to an effective attack or immunity against Lyme disease spirochetes remains to be determined, but it is likely that antibodies alone or in concert with certain lymphocytes halt the erythema migrans rash and the advance of the spirochetes in the skin.

For many people who become infected with Lyme disease spirochetes, this immune response that limits the erythema migrans rash is sufficient to cure them of the infection. The spirochetes have either been completely eliminated from the body or so limited in their spread that they no longer can cause harm. In such cases the only illness the infected person suffers is the rash and some other symptoms that commonly accompany it, which include headache, muscle aches, and tiredness—symptoms that, without the rash, might be called "the flu." As in Julia's case, the temperature may be one or two Fahrenheit degrees above normal, and there may be enlarged lymph glands or nodes near the rash. Some patients have a mild sore throat. Symptoms that are rare during this stage of illness are cough, runny nose, rash on the palms or soles, diarrhea, vomiting, and cramps. If these symptoms occur and there is no rash, the chance that the infection is Lyme disease is minimal.

Werner, Catherine, and Roy had problems with organs and body parts at a distance from the skin. Werner had trouble with his nervous system, Catherine with her joints, and Roy with his heart. In these three people the spirochetes had spread widely from the original site of the infection. Spirochetes accomplish this by first entering the blood from the skin. Once in the bloodstream, they can circulate for one or two weeks. Eventually, antibodies, perhaps aided by lymphocytes, attach to spirochetes in the blood and remove them from the circulation. However, by the time that occurs, some spirochetes have left the blood and entered distant organs. They are able to do this because they can attach themselves to the sides of blood vessels and then penetrate the cells that line veins and arteries. Once they reach the other side of the blood vessels, spirochetes can reside and move in the liquid between cells.

Whether the spirochetes move to and persist in organs and other tissues deep inside the body is one of the critical events that determines whether a person has only erythema migrans or something more serious, as Werner, Catherine, and Roy did. These individuals' immune responses, whether launched with antibodies, lymphocytes, or a combination of both, failed to limit the disease. The spirochetes at some point had entered their blood and spread to other tissues. Even if the immune response eventually removed spirochetes from the blood and skin, the bacteria survived elsewhere. By some method, the spirochetes in these other locations were effectively hidden from the roaming antibodies and lymphocytes.

Complications of Lyme Disease
Infection of the Nervous System

In Werner the spirochetes traveled to the nerves and the brain. These tissues seem to be particularly attractive to Lyme disease spirochetes. The spirochete's motivation—if we can ascribe motivation to a bacterium—in seeking out the brain seems to be that in the brain and some other parts of the nervous system, spirochetes are hidden from the immune response that is so effective in removing them from the blood. In this regard, the Lyme disease spirochetes behave similarly to what might be considered "cousin" spirochetes, those that cause syphilis. In both Lyme disease and syphilis the infection begins in the skin (or, in the case of syphilis alone, the penis, the vagina, the anus, or the mouth). After a period of days or a week, the spirochetes spread from this jumping-off point through the blood to the brain and other tissues. In syphilis it may be months to years until the symptoms of nervous system involvement appear. There is a delay in the onset of neurologic symptoms in Lyme disease, too, lasting from weeks to years.

Werner's problem started with pains in his arm, which he at first blamed on his tennis game. What alarmed him more—and caused him to seek medical attention—was the weakness on one side of his face. One of the nerves that control the facial muscles was affected to the extent that he could not smile or furrow his brow on that side, and his eyelid drooped. This type of nerve paralysis is sometimes called *Bell's palsy*; in Lyme disease the Bell's palsy usually occurs during the summer. Most people with the facial weakness of Lyme disease eventually recover function of the muscles, but some are left with a mild droop on one side of the face. Sometimes both sides of the face are weakened temporarily or permanently.

Paralysis of these muscles is the consequence of inflammation of one of the nerves emerging from the skull, in this case the nerve that connects the brain to the facial muscles. Other such nerves control eye movements or operate the delicate mechanism in the ear. If one or more of these other nerves are involved in Lyme disease, the result may be double vision or difficulty in hearing.

The shooting pain down the arm that Werner experienced was likewise a result of inflammation of the nerves as they emerged from his spinal cord in his neck and back. Other people with nervous system involvement experience pain in the leg or in the trunk. The pain may be accompanied by numbness or loss of sensation in some areas of the body; part of the skin may tingle or feel as if it has "gone to sleep." Some people with Lyme disease neurologic involvement actually experience weakness in their arms or legs. They notice the weakness as they hold a cup or climb a flight of stairs. In some cases the numbness or weakness may occur without being accompanied by pain. Indeed, the severe pains that Werner felt seem to occur less commonly in North America than in Europe. As was true for Bell's palsy, these abnormalities of nerves of the limbs and trunk are not, in isolation, unique to Lyme disease. There may be other medical explanations and, thus, other treatments. Nevertheless, in the context of exposure to the right kind of ticks and a story of a typical skin rash, the odds of Lyme disease are raised.

Because of his medical reading about Lyme disease, perhaps Werner would have been most worried about whether he had a disorder inside the brain itself and not just the nerves emerging from the skull or backbone. He would have been reassured to find out that disease of the brain caused by the Lyme disease spirochete is uncommon. But the prospect of any illness that affects a person's ability to think, concentrate, and remember is chilling.

The symptoms of involvement of the brain during Lyme disease can (rarely) resemble the symptoms of a stroke. There may be profound weakness on one side of body or difficulty in understanding or speaking words. People with these symptoms have spirochetes in their brain, especially around the blood vessels. The presence of the spirochetes causes different types of white blood cells to congregate and water to collect. If there are enough white blood cells and there is enough swelling (from the buildup of water) around the vessels, the passage of blood is blocked or impeded. Deprived of a supply of fresh blood to provide nutrients and removal of wastes, nerve cells cannot function normally. With complete blockage there may even be death of nerve cells. If this happens, thinking, speaking, or the ability to move the limbs may be permanently impaired.

A headache may suggest direct involvement of the brain by the spirochete, but more commonly it is simply a manifestation of the person's nonspecific immune response to infection. In this situation the headache is not caused by spirochetes in the brain itself. Rather it is an effect of the chemicals, including cytokines, released by cells during infection. (The flu-like muscle aches may be another outcome of the body's general response to an infectious disease.) However, if the headache is particularly severe, persists for more than a few days, and is accompanied by neck stiffness, it is possible that the lining surrounding the brain—known as the *meninges*—has become infected. This is a form of *meningitis* (inflammation of the meninges). The lining of the brain swells and stretches, stimulating the nerve endings in the meninges and producing headache pain and neck stiffness. Typically, during meningitis there are more white blood cells in the fluid surrounding the brain.

Infection of the Joints and Tendons

After the spirochetes entered Catherine's blood, they traveled to her joints and months later caused a disabling arthritis in her knee. They may have gone to her brain and nerves, too, but if this happened, Catherine had no symptoms of it. In animals with Lyme disease the spirochetes are commonly found in the joints and the tendons, the tissues that span joints and connect bones.

Catherine's knee pain was disabling but not as severe as the pain caused by rheumatoid arthritis. The swelling was out of proportion to the pain. (In many cases one of the first treatments used to provide pain relief is removal of fluid from the knee with a needle.) The type of arthritis that Catherine had, that is, swelling and pain in one or two large joints, such as the knee, ankle, shoulder, or elbow, usually follows a period earlier in the infection during which several joints and tendons are painful but not usually swollen. Typically the pains migrate from one joint to another, and they come and go. Later, when one or two joints alone are affected, there are weeks in which the pain is intense and other weeks when the person is completely pain free.

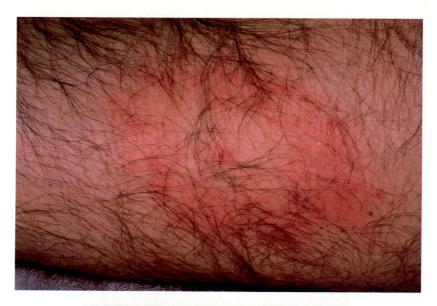

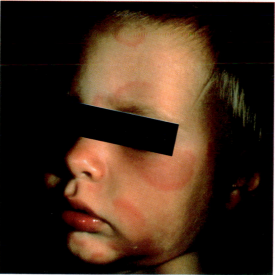

Top: A single erythema migrans rash on the leg. *Bottom:* Multiple rashes of erythema migrans on a child with early disseminated Lyme disease. Some of the rashes are of the same intensity across their diameters; others are darker or lighter in the middle. *Photographs by Jay M. Jones* (top) *and Alan MacDonald* (bottom, *previously published in Alan G. Barbour, "Laboratory Aspects of Lyme Borreliosis,"* Clinical Microbiology Reviews *1 [1988]: 400).*

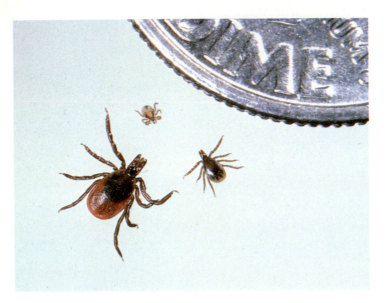

Next to a dime are the larva *(smallest)*, nymph *(intermediate-sized)*, and adult female *(largest)* of *Ixodes scapularis,* the deer tick of the central and eastern United States. *Photograph courtesy of Russell Johnson.*

Sometimes the temporomandibular joint, the place where the lower jaw is connected to the skull, is painful. The small joints of the hands and feet are usually not involved at any stage of Lyme disease.

Whether a more chronic and disabling arthritis develops may be determined by the person's genetic background. There are certain genes, known as MHC genes, which a person inherits from his or her parents and which may put the person at higher risk of severe, long-lasting arthritis during Lyme disease. The same genes also increase a person's risk of developing rheumatoid arthritis. This is one reason many researchers think that if scientists can reach an understanding of the cause of arthritis in Lyme disease, they may discover important clues for understanding rheumatoid arthritis and other disabling disorders of the joints as well. The infectious organism that causes the arthritis of Lyme disease is known. If a bacterium or virus triggers rheumatoid arthritis, it has yet to be unequivocally identified.

It is not yet known why some people with MHC genes develop a more severe form of Lyme arthritis and one that is more difficult to treat. In rheumatoid arthritis the person may mount an immune response against his or her own tissues and cells. This type of inappropriate, potentially damaging immune response is called *autoimmunity*. There is some circumstantial evidence that autoimmunity occurs in certain people with Lyme disease. One piece of evidence is the finding that some antibodies against the Lyme disease spirochete also react with human tissues. Because antibodies can take only a limited number of shapes, some of them by chance may bind or fit with cells and tissues of the person or animal in whose body they were created, as well as with a part of the invading microorganism. When this occurs, a molecule or other structure in those cells and tissues seems to the antibody or lymphocyte to be identical to part of the microorganism. The bacterium or virus is said to mimic a substance in the person or animal it infects.

Normally there are effective checks to prevent these injurious antibodies and lymphocytes from proliferating and then, in higher numbers, causing trouble. Otherwise people would constantly be producing immune responses to themselves. But some human systems aren't able to prevent some of these harmful antibodies and lymphocytes from increasing in numbers. The bacteria or viruses that the immune attack was directed against may be dead, but the immune response continues to act against the person's own tissues.

Infection of the Heart

Roy's collapse on the street landed him in a hospital's intensive care unit. If his heart rate had been much slower, he might have died from this complication of Lyme disease. Deaths as a direct result of the disease are rare—perhaps fewer than ten have occurred in the world. But when a fatality does occur, it likely is attributable to involvement of the heart in Lyme disease.

Animals with the Lyme disease infection frequently have spirochetes in their heart. Spirochetes seem to preferentially settle in the heart, as well as in the joints and nervous system, in people as well as in animals. The microorganisms enter the muscles of the heart and there produce inflammation. The white blood cells increase in numbers, and the spaces between cells swell with fluid. This inflammation of the heart's muscles can reduce the strength of the heart's contractions, and in this condition the heart cannot sustain the same load it normally would.

If the inflammation is in the conduction system for the heartbeat, the impulses are slowed or blocked. The electrical message for the heartbeat, which starts in the upper part of the heart, cannot reach the lower heart, where the pumping action is strongest. The lower heart has a backup conduction system that comes into play if the impulses cannot get through to it. But the backup's intrinsic rate of beating is much lower than that of the normal control system—thirty to forty beats per minute rather than sixty to eighty. At rates this slow, the heart may not be able to pump enough blood to supply the vital organs, such as the brain. The symptoms of slowed or blocked electrical messages in the heart include fainting, or a feeling of light-headedness that might be relieved by lying down.

Other Manifestations of Lyme Disease

The nervous system, the joints, and the heart—these are the organs and tissues commonly affected by the spirochete when it spreads in the blood. But other parts of the body may be involved, too: the eyes, for example, and the muscles of the limbs and trunk, as well as the liver. One of the indications that the spirochete has spread is the appearance of additional erythema migrans rashes. These usually appear within several days after the first skin rash. There may be only one additional red patch or many. The patient usually also feels sick with fever, headache, and general achiness. It is not uncommon for multiple skin rashes and involvement of the nervous system, heart, or joints to occur at the same time.

When one or both eyes are affected, there may be a change in vision and an increased sensitivity to light. Redness of the "whites" of the eyes is usually not by itself a sign of Lyme disease; there are many other explanations for this symptom. When the muscles are inflamed, there may be soreness and tenderness that is greater than the generalized achiness accompanying an infection. Again, if muscle tenderness and pain is the only symptom, Lyme disease would be an unlikely explanation. Among the possible explanations of muscle pain are many that would rank higher than Lyme disease, even in areas where the infection is common. If, however, the muscle pain had started a few weeks after the appearance of a targetlike skin rash, then Lyme disease would climb far up the list of the possibilities for a diagnosis.

Early studies of Lyme disease patients in North America revealed minor abnormalities in their blood. These abnormalities, discovered during testing, were of some use to physicians in making the diagnosis if their suspicion of Lyme disease was already high. But the abnormalities were not specific for Lyme disease—that is, there were other medical conditions that produced similar abnormalities in the blood. Since the discovery of the Lyme disease spirochete and the availability of a specific diagnostic test, these blood abnormalities have assumed less importance. Nevertheless, the types of abnormalities that were observed provided additional insight into how the spirochete affects people.

What physicians found was evidence of mild liver damage and increased production of all antibodies, not just the ones against the spirochete. The liver damage discovered in a minority of patients was detectable only by the blood tests—physicians discovered no evidence of a problem with the liver simply by talking to or examining the patient. This situation, in which an abnormality in a blood test of liver function is present without evidence of significant disease of the liver, occurs frequently in medicine. It probably results from the liver's tendency to release its enzymes and other proteins into the bloodstream after relatively minor injuries. In any case, the finding of higher levels than normal of liver enzymes in the blood is not uncommon during Lyme disease and does not usually indicate a serious problem with that organ. Only a few patients with Lyme disease have had liver inflammation to the point of developing true hepatitis.

The increase in many types of antibodies in the blood is more difficult to assess. With some infections it is common for antibodies to be produced not only against the microorganism that caused the infection but also against other invaders. The presence of the microorganism seems to turn on the production of various kinds of antibodies, even those that would not be protective. It's as if, in response to a general alarm, all the troops are called up instead of only the handful of specially trained soldiers called for in the situation. This phenomenon also occurs in some autoimmune diseases, such as lupus erythematosus and rheumatoid arthritis. In fact, as we will consider later in more detail, some of the extra antibodies produced in autoimmune diseases such as lupus may be directed against parts of the Lyme disease spirochete, giving a false test result. For the most part, in Lyme disease the antibodies are usually not increased to levels that would be expected to produce problems.

What Part of the Body Isn't Affected by Lyme Disease?

After this litany of the troubles caused by the Lyme disease spirochete, it may seem that no part of the body remains uninvolved when this infection occurs—but that's not so. Most of the body's organs and tissues—for instance, the lungs, the kidneys, the bones, the pancreas, the gall bladder, and the intestinal tract from the esophagus to the anus—are rarely if ever affected in Lyme disease. Indeed, if there is evidence of infection or other abnormality in these other body locations in humans, it indicates that the disorder is either not

Lyme disease or includes something else in addition to Lyme disease. In Lyme disease, too, there is seldom any abnormality of the glands that produce hormones, such as the thyroid and adrenal glands. Lyme disease does not appear to increase the risk of a heart attack from blockage of an artery. It does not cause cancer, diabetes, hemorrhoids, hyperthyroidism, leukemia, osteoporosis, psoriasis, heartburn, or a hernia. There is no evidence that it causes a condition like AIDS or other forms of serious depression of the immune system.

Although Lyme disease can affect the brain and the rest of the nervous system, studies have confirmed that the Lyme disease spirochete does not cause multiple sclerosis (often called "MS") or amyotrophic lateral sclerosis, otherwise known as "ALS" or "Lou Gehrig's disease." That is not to say that Lyme disease can't sometimes look like these other neurologic disorders, especially multiple sclerosis in the early stages, or that a Lyme disease infection may not worsen a case of multiple sclerosis. Rather, there is no convincing evidence that multiple sclerosis or Lou Gehrig's disease, as they are currently defined, are causally related to Lyme disease. This may be bad news for people suffering from those conditions: if a spirochete were the cause in either case, there would be hope for a cure with antibiotics. But at least the knowledge that multiple sclerosis and Lou Gehrig's disease are not caused by a spirochete means that researchers can turn to more productive lines of research on the causes of these disorders. Moreover, the similarities between Lyme disease of the brain and multiple sclerosis may yet yield clues to the real cause or causes of MS.

Can Lyme Disease Be Passed to the Fetus during Pregnancy?

The similarities between Lyme disease and syphilis have been mentioned. One of the feared consequences of infection with *Treponema pallidum*, the spirochete that causes syphilis, is transmission of the spirochete to an infected woman's developing fetus. As the rate of syphilis has climbed in the United States in the last decade, there have been many more cases of congenital syphilis in children born to women infected with *Treponema pallidum*. This can result in tragedy, because these babies are sometimes born with malformed faces and bones or mental retardation.

To date, the number of cases in which the fetus contracted Lyme disease while in the womb has been very small. Even if the fetus does become infected with the spirochete during a woman's pregnancy, there is little evidence that this very often leads to miscarriages, still-births, or babies with internal or external deformities. If Lyme disease during pregnancy does cause stillbirths and sick or abnormal babies, it does this rarely enough that the effect cannot be noticed in studies comparing areas with high and low risks of Lyme disease. These findings should by no means lead to complacency about Lyme disease in women of child-bearing age: it's important to take extra precautions to prevent all kinds of infections in pregnant women. One infected newborn is one too many. Still, it is reassuring that, among the children of women infected with *B. burgdorferi*, congenital Lyme disease seems to occur at a much lower rate than does congenital syphilis among the children of women who are infected with the latter disease.

Are People with Lower Resistance at Special Risk of Complications from Lyme Disease?

Another group of people who might be expected to do poorly with Lyme disease are those with lowered resistance to infection. If, as we have seen, the immune system can ultimately control the infection in many if not all people, then shouldn't those with defective immune systems be at a higher risk of infection and more serious disease? People with AIDS come to mind, as do people with transplants or cancer who are on drugs that suppress the immune system. We could also include the very young and older people. The infant immune system is not as effective as the immune system in the older child and adult, and after a person passes the age of seventy or so the immune system loses some of its ability to thwart infections and check cancer growth.

Perhaps surprisingly, there is neither a discernibly higher rate of Lyme disease infection nor a greater risk of severe Lyme disease among people with AIDS or those on medications that reduce their ability to fight infection. With AIDS and most immunity-suppressing drugs the principal deficiency is in the cells that respond to infection, and the antibodies are less severely affected. Studies of Lyme disease in animals indicate that antibodies are more important than are disease-fighting cells in controlling this spirochete infection. Thus, as long as a person has the ability to make antibodies, it is likely that infection can be controlled. Indeed, a reduction in the cellular part of the immune response may actually lower the risk of arthritis. As we have seen, the cells that some patients send to the joints may cause more harm than good. Very young and very old people may have deficiencies in producing antibodies. But people in these age groups have a low risk of Lyme disease because they are less likely to be out of doors and thus are less likely to be exposed to ticks.

What Happens When Dogs and Other Domestic Animals Get Lyme Disease?

The ticks that carry the Lyme disease spirochetes bite pets as well their owners. Among all the domestic animals at risk of infection, dogs appear to contract the disease most often. In some areas of the United States, the majority of dogs in the community appear to have been infected with the Lyme disease spirochete. Like people, most dogs do not get very sick from the infection, but some develop a lameness in the legs that is the equivalent of the arthritis of Lyme disease. There is pain, warmth, and swelling of one or more of the affected joints. The dog refuses to bear weight on the limb with the sore joint. The lameness may be accompanied by fever, lethargy, listlessness, and loss of appetite, and the arthritis may come and go over several months. As with people, the onset of the arthritis may not occur until weeks to months after the dog's exposure to ticks. Some dogs also develop disease of their kidneys, a complication that has not been observed in humans. All breeds of dog appear to be susceptible to infection with the spirochete. Indeed, dogs generally are at a higher risk of infection than are people. Dogs, especially those allowed to run free, have a higher exposure to ticks than most people do.

There is evidence that cats, cows, horses, and sheep can be infected with the Lyme disease spirochete, but the information on infections in these other animals is not extensive. The most compelling data exist on infections of horses. There are reports of lameness, with tender, swollen joints, in some horses living in areas where Lyme disease is common.

Overview of the Infection

When physicians and nurses speak of the clinical features of a disease, they mean those aspects that can be discovered by talking to the patient, examining the patient, and performing laboratory tests and other technical procedures, such as an x-ray or electrocardiogram. The ecological or preventative aspects of Lyme disease are another matter. This chapter focused on the clinical features.

Given that there are exceptions to almost every categorization scheme, we can still discern that symptomatic infection with *B. burgdorferi* evolves over time with a certain pattern. The course of the infection can be divided into *localized early infection; disseminated early infection;* and *late infection,* which is also called *chronic Lyme disease.* These three designations roughly correspond to time periods, measured from the start of infection, of days, weeks, and months, respectively. This temporal pattern to the illness can be an important clue that someone has Lyme disease: many patients with *B. burgdorferi* infection do not present with all the classic manifestations of Lyme disease, but one can still discern a waxing and waning of an illness lasting weeks to months.

Localized early infection is an erythema migrans rash limited to the site of a tick bite. There may be swelling of lymph glands near the bite, as well as generalized achiness and a headache. The patient's temperature is only mildly elevated if it is elevated at all. From a localized infection, the untreated patient's illness may progress to the disseminated form, either directly or after a temporary period of well-being. Disseminated early infection is characterized by one or more of the following symptoms: (1) two or more erythema migrans rashes, (2) migrating pains of the joints and tendons, (3) headache with stiff neck, (4) Bell's palsy, (5) pains down the arms or legs, (6) multiple enlarged lymph glands, (6) slowing of the heart, (7) sore throat, (8) changes in the vision, (9) temperatures of 100°F to 102°F, and (10) severe fatigue.

Patients with disseminated early infection may receive medical attention and treatment. If they do not, or if the treatment is inadequate, months later the patients may begin to have one or more symptoms and signs of late infection. The most typical manifestations of late infection in North America are arthritis of one or two large joints, disabling disorders of the brain and spinal cord, and loss of sensation in the arms or legs. This stage of infection with *B. burgdorferi* is harder to define and to distinguish from other medical conditions. Chronic Lyme disease also has to be differentiated from symptoms that linger after otherwise adequate therapy of early *B. burgdorferi* infection.

The problem of chronic Lyme disease—its definition, diagnosis, and management—is discussed further in Chapters 5 to 8. Before returning to these and other clinical aspects of Lyme disease, though, we consider the infection from a perspective that includes its history, ecology, and public health aspects.

2

The Enigma
of an Emerging Disease

Although Lyme disease takes its name from a town in Connecticut, what we now recognize as an infection by a spirochete was first recorded in Europe around the turn of the century. At that time, and for many years after, the disease was called *erythema chronicum migrans*. European physicians noted the association of this distinctive skin rash with a prior tick bite. Thereafter, a peculiar disorder of the nervous system, called, among other names, Bannwarth's syndrome, was also linked to exposure to the same types of ticks in Europe and Russia. Some of the patients with this syndrome had suffered from erythema chronicum migrans before their pains and weaknesses began.

Not until the 1960s was the skin rash observed in North America. But physicians in the United States were the first to realize that disorders of the joints and the heart were part of the same complex of tick-borne infection. Gradually, the disease that had been known variously as erythema chronicum migrans, Bannwarth's syndrome, and "erythema migrans disease" came to be called Lyme disease or, in some places, Lyme borreliosis. When similar infections were found more recently in Asia, they were called Lyme disease.

Lyme disease is now a common infectious disease in parts of North America, Europe, and Russia. In these regions it is the infection most frequently carried by insects or by ticks (both of which are members of the animal group known as *arthropods*). Reports of the disease in these areas outnumber reports of other arthropod-borne diseases such as malaria, Rocky Mountain spotted fever, yellow fever, typhus, arboviral encephalitis, relapsing fever, and Chagas's disease. In the United States, Lyme disease is more commonly reported than Legionnaire's disease and toxic shock syndrome, other diseases discovered about the same time. It occurs more often than measles, mumps, polio, tetanus, diphtheria, and whooping cough, all of which are controlled by vaccines in the United States and Europe. For the entire country, Lyme disease is somewhat less common than tuberculosis and far less common than influenza, strep throat, food poisoning, and gonorrhea.

Because of increases in the numbers of cases of Lyme disease and in the disease's geographic spread, Lyme disease has been listed (along with AIDS, hantavirus infections, and tuberculosis, among other infections) as one of the world's "emerging diseases." Its new prominence as an actual and perceived health problem in North America can be traced to some specific ecological and biological factors, such as the reforestation of parts of North America and increases in deer populations. We can easily observe that forests have regained some lands that were formerly devoted to farming, and that deer, once close to eradication in the northeastern United States, are numerous enough to be a nuisance in the suburbs. Ticks that carry the infection have also been found in some areas, such as northern Sweden, that used to be too cold for ticks to survive in, a finding that suggests a regional if not a global change in climate.

But there are also social factors in Lyme disease's emergence as a public and individual concern. These include value changes—changes in what much of society considers important. For instance, a desire to live near wildlife, combined with a reluctance to apply pesticides in the environment, increases people's chances of contact with insects and ticks. People are very active players in regional and global ecological transformations: in fact, the major cause of reforestation and increasing deer populations in North America is neither a climatic shift nor a natural decline in large animal predators, but rather, human activity.

The amount of attention paid to Lyme disease is determined as much by media decisions as by the actual threat the disease poses to people. Among infectious diseases, Lyme disease has ranked only behind AIDS as a hot media topic over the last several years. Hepatitis, syphilis, and some other infectious diseases are more common than Lyme disease, but they are not perceived as a significant health threat by much of the public, in part because the media have not focused as much attention on these diseases. There are few newspaper or magazine profiles of people coping with syphilis, in contrast to dozens of such profiles of people with Lyme disease. A significant aspect of such media decisions is their effect on the public's understanding of disease processes, including the prevention, transmission, prevalence, and treatment of disease. Most people know that they can get AIDS from unprotected sex, for example, but few know that they are more likely to get a debilitating form of hepatitis from such activity.

The phenomenon of Lyme disease includes not only the thousands of people actually infected with the Lyme disease spirochete but also the equal or greater number of people who have been inaccurately diagnosed as having the infection. What these people have is a disabling illness and deserves attention, but the cause of illness in many of these cases appears to be something other than the spirochete.

Assumptions and Definitions

Lyme disease remains an enigma in many respects, and much remains to be learned from further study and research. At present even the definition of the disease is controversial, so it's easy to see why discussions about its treatment and prevention create a stir. The debates and areas of ignorance are not avoided in this book. Still, if every point of view were presented here in depth, this book would become very cumbersome. To avoid this, some assumptions had to be made. For example, a decision was made to use the term *Lyme disease* instead of *Lyme borreliosis* throughout the book. The rationale for this decision was simple: more people use the former term than the latter.

Two other assumptions were made for this and the next chapter's description of Lyme disease in human populations and in nature: for the presentation of the natural history or ecology of Lyme disease, it is assumed that the disease results from infection with a tick-borne spirochete, and that in the absence of evidence of exposure to ticks that carry the spirochete the diagnosis of Lyme disease cannot be made. Later chapters review the debate about the validity of this assumption.

Another assumption concerns the name of the bacterium that causes the disease. Throughout the book the microorganism that produces Lyme disease is called *Borrelia burgdorferi*. This was the name given to the first isolates of the bacteria from ticks, animals, and people in the United States and Europe. Some experts, however, suggest that the group of bacteria included under the umbrella name *Borrelia burgdorferi* should be divided into at least four different species. At present the three other proposed species (besides *Borrelia burgdorferi*) are *Borrelia afzelii*, *Borrelia garinii*, and *Borrelia japonica*. Other experts dispute the need for this species subdivision. To someone outside the field of bacteria classification this dispute may seem like the argument about how many angels can dance on the head of a pin—in other words, of little practical importance. Because in fact the advantage of having four species names instead of one is not yet obvious, and because the name *Borrelia burgdorferi* is already widely accepted and known, I use that name in this book for all bacteria that are known to cause Lyme disease. If distinctions between Lyme disease bacteria are important for understanding such matters as vaccines or diagnostic tests, they will be presented as differences between *strains* of B. *burgdorferi* and not as differences between species. Strains are like different members of the same extended family.

A Strange Disease Outbreak in Connecticut

Professional, media, and public awareness of Lyme disease in the United States began to increase in the late 1970s and has continued to do so through the 1980s and 1990s. Erythema migrans, the characteristic skin rash of the infection, had been described in North American residents in the medical literature since 1970, but because these early cases were sporadic and were reported from different parts of the country, they drew little attention. Then, in 1975, an unusual disease outbreak occurred among residents of Lyme, Connecticut. This outbreak was covered in the newspapers and on television newscasts, and Lyme disease has been in the news ever since.

Lyme and adjoining towns are located near Long Island Sound and the Atlantic Ocean. Founded in the seventeenth century, they still have town squares of grass, with white-steepled churches. Around the town centers are forested areas, and many of the older houses sit on lots of an acre or more. Lyme and similar towns, while retaining much of their village character and charm, are often commuter communities of nearby cities, such as New Haven. Most of the residents of these towns are middle class or more affluent, and unlike residents of Lyme of three hundred years ago, most of the town's present-day citizens work outside the town.

The investigation of the disease outbreak in Lyme began when Polly Morray and Judith Mensch called the Connecticut state health department. Each of these women had a child who had been diagnosed as having arthritis—that is, swelling and pain of one or more joints. The two mothers were also aware of other children, as well as adults, in town who had recently begun having symptoms of joint disease. While arthritis is not unusual in older adults, it is extremely uncommon in children. For several children in the same town to have this diagnosis was more than simple coincidence or bad luck could account for.

The health department began its investigation and at an early point contacted Allen Steere and his colleagues at Yale University, in New Haven. Steere was beginning his training in rheumatology, the medical subspecialty focusing on joints, muscles, and connective tissue; and before that, he had gained experience in the investigation of disease outbreaks as a Public Health Service officer. He had the right background, and he was in the right place at the right time. More important, though, he perceived that this outbreak could be something important and that it deserved full attention. One reason it was important was that it might provide a clue about the infectious agent or environmental toxin that was responsible for arthritis (the cause of rheumatoid arthritis has been sought for years).

Steere and his fellow investigators carried out several studies of the arthritis outbreak around Lyme. Additional cases were identified, and the people with the disease, as well as members of their families and other people without the disease, were questioned about risk factors for the disease. The unaffected people served as a *control* group for the investigation. If an exposure to any one particular thing was more common among people with the disease than among people without the disease, then that thing might be an important clue to the cause of the outbreak. As a fanciful example, consider that if nine of the eleven people with symptoms ate bananas but only two of the twelve "controls" did—a difference unlikely to occur by chance alone—then banana consumption would be an important lead to follow up on.

One critical early observation was the association between the arthritis and a prior skin rash. At Yale, a visiting physician from Europe pointed out that the skin rash was similar to erythema migrans, a frequently encountered disease from tick bites in northern Europe. On the basis of the distribution and seasonal timing of the cases, and the noted association of arthritis and skin rash, field studies and surveys of patients were carried out.

What Steere and his collaborators found has essentially been confirmed in other locales, including sites in Europe, Russia, and Asia. The information gained from their studies, and studies by others, is presented in this chapter. The essential findings of the first group of studies of the "Lyme arthritis" phenomenon were these:

First, the disease was seasonal, being most common in the summer and least common in the middle of winter. In geographic areas with cold winters, such as Connecticut, this finding suggested either a summer virus or an infection carried by an insect or tick. Some viruses are more common in the winter in temperate climates; others are more likely to spread in the warmer months. (Before a polio vaccine was available, for example, poliovirus infections were most common in the summer months in the United States.)

Second, the disease did not seem to spread from one person in a family to another. This would not be typical of the summer viruses, which characteristically are spread from person to person, especially among those in the same household. When this mode of transmission was excluded, the spotlight was focused on the involvement of arthropods in the outbreak.

Third, the disease was much more common on one side of the Connecticut River, which bisects the state, than on the other. There was a good correlation with the frequency of a certain tick now named *Ixodes scapularis*. This type of tick had been implicated in carrying a rare blood parasite but otherwise was considered harmless in the United States. But the evidence was there: the tick was most prevalent on the side of the river with the most cases of Lyme arthritis. When questioned, some people remembered having had a tick bite before the symptoms of arthritis started.

The Discovery of the Infectious Agent

With the inclusion of a skin rash and disorders of the nervous system and heart in the case definition, "Lyme arthritis" became "Lyme disease." When the broader definition was applied, more cases were found, not only in Connecticut but in adjoining states and the upper Midwest as well. The evidence strongly suggested that Lyme disease was an infectious disease spread by ticks, but the identity of the infectious agent remained a mystery. There are many varieties of ticks, and different ticks carry different agents: viruses, bacteria, protozoa, or even small worms. If the Lyme disease agent was a virus—a microorganism that cannot exist on its own and instead is heavily dependent on the cell that it infects—it might be identified in a culture grown in the laboratory. When viruses are cultivated in the laboratory they are grown in mammalian cells living in artificial solutions that mimic conditions inside the body. These artificial solutions are called *culture media*.

If it was a bacterium—a one-celled organism that is complete unto itself—there was the chance that it could be seen by a common microscope and even isolated in standard hospital laboratories in culture media. Some bacteria, however, are restricted to the insides of other cells for life and cannot be grown outside of cells. In this respect these cell-bound bacteria are like viruses and need special conditions to be grown and identified in the laboratory. Other bacteria, even if they are not limited to the insides of cells, have unique requirements for growth. Since there are thousands of supplements that can be added to the culture medium used in growing bacteria, choosing the one that works for a particular bacterium is sometimes a matter of luck.

Erythema migrans had been suspected to be an infectious disease in Europe long before the outbreak in Lyme. One courageous if foolhardy investigator produced the disease in others by injecting some tissue from a patient's erythema migrans lesion into their skin. This was strong evidence that the disease was transmissible. Among the different possible agents for Lyme disease, bacteria were highest on the list. European physicians were treating patients with medicines that would be effective against bacteria. But the evidence from Europe in favor of a bacterial agent for erythema migrans was not without its flaws, and consequently was not accepted at first in the United States.

The investigators of Lyme disease in Connecticut and erythema migrans in Europe searched for the Lyme disease agent itself, and for its tracks, both in the incriminated ticks and in patients. Many known viruses and bacteria were considered, but none of them could be implicated with any confidence. It appeared that whatever was causing Lyme disease was something new. The search narrowed to bacteria when the researchers in Connecticut and their colleagues confirmed from their own studies that patients with Lyme disease improved with antibiotics. Bacteria, but not viruses, protozoans, or fungi, are affected by the antibiotics the physicians used.

At this time, by now 1981, another group of investigators became involved—by chance rather than by design—in the search. These scientists were based at Montana's Rocky Mountain Laboratories, a branch of the National Institutes of Health. The laboratories were far away from any known Lyme disease cases, but they had for several decades been a center for studies of the infectious diseases carried by ticks and insects.

One of the experts on a variety of tick-borne diseases at the Montana laboratories was Willy Burgdorfer. Burgdorfer, when he first came to the Rocky Mountain Laboratories thirty years previously from his native Switzerland, had studied a certain kind of spirochete that is passed between people and other animals by ticks. But he soon was discouraged by administrators in Washington from working in this area because these spirochetes and relapsing fever, the disease they caused, were not judged to be important for human health in the United States. In more recent years he had focused his work on Rocky Mountain spotted fever, a frequently fatal infection passed by ticks.

The history of the government's lack of enthusiasm for research on relapsing fever was not known to me, though, when I began studies on this disease in 1980 at the Rocky Mountain Laboratories. Over the succeeding months I learned to grow these spirochetes in a special medium invented several years previously by Richard Kelly, and more recently improved by Herbert Stoenner, one of the scientists at the Montana laboratory. Further tinkering by me led to what came to be called "BSK medium" for growing this class of bacteria.

In the fall of 1981 Burgdorfer received some ticks to examine from his colleague Jorge Benach, a scientist in New York. The two investigators were carrying out a study of Rocky Mountain spotted fever on Long Island, an area known to have both Rocky Mountain spotted fever and Lyme disease. Burgdorfer studied the ticks by looking at their contents under a microscope, a difficult procedure performed by few other scientists. One day while doing this he saw something that should not have been there: the long, wavy form of a spirochete. Spirochetes had never been seen in the *Ixodes* group of ticks before. They were only known to occur in a completely separate group of ticks that had very different habits. He opened up other ticks from Long Island and saw the same spiral-shaped bacteria in many of them, too. Burgdorfer realized the possible relationship with Lyme disease: spirochetes are a type of bacteria that would be killed by the antibiotics used to treat Lyme disease.

My own involvement in Lyme disease began at that time. Burgdorfer gave me some of the ticks, and I grew the spirochetes for the first time in the laboratory. Using the newly cultivated spirochetes as the basis of a diagnostic test, Burgdorfer and I examined the blood of several patients from Long Island who had Lyme disease. A primary care physician, Edgar Grunwaldt, whose medical practice was located at the northern tip of Long Island, had, with great foresight, saved frozen samples of blood from his patients. In the laboratory we found that the blood from Grunwaldt's patients showed evidence that they had been exposed to the new spirochete. Blood from healthy people living elsewhere did not have the same type of reaction. It looked as if the cause of Lyme disease had been identified.

Further proof came when the same spirochetes found in the ticks were recovered from patients with Lyme disease, first by Steere and

Benach and their colleagues in the United States, and subsequently by investigators in Europe. Ticks from the Midwest and California, and from Europe, Russia, China, and Japan, had the same type of spirochetes, by that time named *Borrelia burgdorferi*. These discoveries also showed that erythema migrans and the tick-borne nerve disorder in Europe were the same infection that had been called Lyme disease in North America.

Since that time the term *Lyme disease*, or its variant *Lyme borreliosis*, has become the accepted name for this infection worldwide. In other languages *disease* or *borreliosis* may be replaced by equivalent words, but *Lyme* comes through, as the example of *Laimo* in Lithuanian shows. Patients in California, Switzerland, Russia, and Japan all use the name of a Connecticut town as a name for their illness. A misconception is that *Lyme* refers to a person, perhaps the first patient with the disease, or its discoverer. Under that mistaken assumption, Lyme disease has become for many people "Lyme's disease" or plain "Lyme's."

Case Counting

Over the last few years about ten thousand cases of Lyme disease have been reported annually to the public health authorities in the United States. In 1994 the number was more than thirteen thousand. The number of reported cases of Lyme disease in the United States rose rapidly in the 1980s to the present levels. In part this increase in case numbers is due to an increased frequency of infection, but the higher numbers are also attributable to a better accounting of cases: during this period states began to list Lyme disease as one of the "reportable" diseases for public health purposes. Also, more physicians became aware of the condition, so that what might have been thought in the past to be a severe reaction to a tick bite was now recognized as Lyme disease by the physician.

Even as the number of cases being reported to the health agencies was increasing, however, there was a growing realization that many of the reported cases did not represent *B. burgdorferi* infection. One state listed hundreds of cases of "Lyme disease" in one year, until public health investigators determined that the risk of acquiring the disease in that state was very low and that it would have been impossible for that many cases of Lyme disease to have occurred. There followed a toughening of standards for what would be officially listed as a case of the disease. The rise in numbers of actual infections and in disease awareness was counterbalanced by stricter definitions for case reporting of Lyme disease.

How accurately does the official count reflect the true state of Lyme disease in the United States? There are two ways of looking at that question. The first is to ask whether the *case definition*—that is, the criterion for diagnosis—used for reporting purposes is overly strict. As stated earlier in this chapter, this is a controversial question, both sides of which will be discussed in greater detail elsewhere in this book. Instead, what we're asking here is whether there is an undercount of cases of Lyme disease even by today's official definition. In other words, are there still large numbers of cases unnoticed, unreported, and consequently uncounted by governmental health agencies?

The implications of an undercount are considerable, since to a large extent the amount of research monies devoted to a particular disease is determined by the *incidence*, or yearly frequency, of new cases of that disease in the population. For chronic diseases (that is, diseases lasting more than a few weeks or months), the other measure of importance for funding purposes is *prevalence*, or the proportion of people in the population with the disease at any given time. There are more research grants available for cancer, diabetes, AIDS, or heart disease than for bubonic plague (or Lyme disease, for that matter). Cancer, diabetes, AIDS, and heart disease not only have a high incidence, they are also highly prevalent. Many people are newly diagnosed with one of these conditions each year, and those patients still living will have the disease in the next year and possibly the year after that. The prevalence count of heart disease is the total number of living people with that disorder; the original diagnosis may have been made last week or twenty years earlier.

Contrast this with bubonic plague, in some eras and some parts of the world a very common and deadly disease. At present there are only a handful of new cases of plague each year in the United States;

the incidence of plague is very low. If a person is unfortunate enough to be infected with the plague bacterium, the illness is comparatively brief, ending in either cure or death. The prevalence of plague, therefore, is even lower than the incidence. Thus, what was historically one of the most significant killers of people is now relegated to the status of a minor disease in the United States; for now, Lyme disease is in the ascendancy in plague's wake.

The number of reported cases of a disease also has an impact on the plans and budgets of governmental and nonprofit agencies whose mission is the prevention of disease. The resources devoted to the prevention of AIDS or cancer through educational measures and tracking efforts are much greater than those devoted to the prevention of bubonic plague. The pharmaceutical and diagnostic test industries also look at the incidence and prevalence of disease. Business decisions about whether to develop a product for treatment or diagnosis are driven by estimates of what the market will be. A new drug treatment or vaccine may cost a company upwards of $100 million for development, testing, and marketing. Obviously, stockholders would not be pleased if such an effort were devoted to an infrequent disease, no matter how noble the intention. One of the reasons for the delay in development of reliable diagnostic tests for Lyme disease was the underestimation by large companies of the numbers of people who were being tested for evidence of *B. burgdorferi* infection.

Experience with other infections and diseases that are formally tallied by state and federal health agencies suggests that for every reported case of a given infectious disease there is a variable number of unreported cases. The ratio varies according to the degree of incentive for reporting and the perceived threat to the public health. For instance, the count of AIDS cases that is reported to state health departments and the federal Centers for Disease Control and Prevention is probably close to the actual number of people who are first diagnosed as having AIDS each year. One reason is that physicians recognize the importance of reporting a disease, such as AIDS or tuberculosis, that can be passed from one person to another. Further incentives are that people become eligible for certain disability benefits once they have been reported to have AIDS, and may possibly receive free health care once active tuberculosis has been reported. Of course, there are people with AIDS or tuberculosis who are not included in these numbers, but that is usually because they have not yet reached medical attention.

There has been less incentive from a public health perspective to accurately track Lyme disease than AIDS. For one thing, Lyme disease is rarely fatal: only a few deaths are attributable to the disease in the entire world. For another, *B. burgdorferi* infection is not spread between people, either directly or indirectly. People cannot get Lyme disease—unlike AIDS and some forms of hepatitis—from their sexual partners. Nor can they get it from eating food prepared by someone else, or from breathing air contaminated by someone's cough. Because it is acquired from a tick and not from another person, it is not likely to produce the case numbers that AIDS and such readily communicable diseases as influenza have. *B. burgdorferi* infection does not travel quickly through a community in the way that cholera or a cold virus can, and accordingly there has been little fear that Lyme disease will get quickly out of hand.

For some time, governmental agencies and other institutions did not recognize that many people were being diagnosed as or suspected of having an active *B. burgdorferi* infection when in fact they did not. These cases don't appear in the official tallies because they generally do not meet the strict case definition for Lyme disease. Nevertheless, these patients receive medical services and care, including lengthy and expensive treatments with intravenous antibiotics. Many or most of these people are disabled to some extent: they are not able to make their lives as active and fulfilling as they would wish. In a sense, they have chronic illnesses that, like heart disease, persist from one year to the next.

The media recognized this phenomenon early. Though an argument could be made that the public's interest has been fed by the frequent articles and reports on the infection, there doesn't seem to be any question that the public is fascinated by articles on Lyme disease. Stories in newspapers and magazines and on television frequently focused on people whose illnesses were far from consistent with *B. burgdorferi* infection yet who were described as having the disease.

While governmental and academic institutions, in their determinations and studies of "real" cases of the infection, were treating these dubious cases as so much noise, the media, with a few exceptions, were not concerned about such diagnostic subtleties. If a person said that he or she had Lyme disease, the media usually accepted this diagnosis without question. Why, common sense asks, would someone say that he or she had a disease when in fact he or she did not?

In trying to answer the question of how many cases of Lyme disease are actually occurring, we have no choice but to accept the official number and apply an adjustment factor to correct for underreporting. Lyme disease would be underreported if only a fraction of the physicians who made the diagnosis sent in a report of the case to their local or state health department during a given year. Judging from the reporting of other infectious diseases comparable to Lyme disease, we can adjust the number of cases upwards roughly fivefold. This estimate is also based on the findings of surveys of individual communities, in which researchers actively looked for people with Lyme disease. Having made that correction, we can estimate that the total number of people who get Lyme disease each year in the United States may be as high as fifty thousand to sixty thousand. This is two to four people for every ten thousand.

Geography and the Risk of Lyme Disease

These thousands of cases of Lyme disease are not distributed randomly or equally across the United States but, rather, are concentrated in certain regions and absent in others. In this respect Lyme disease is not like schizophrenia, which occurs with a certain likelihood to people wherever they may live or whatever their geographic origins. Among all common diseases in the United States and Europe, Lyme disease is unusual in the degree to which its occurrence is determined by location. The frequency of other diseases may be influenced to some degree by geographic area, but the influence is usually not so dramatic as in the case of Lyme disease. Skin cancers, for example, are more common in residents of Southern California than among people who live in Alaska, but Alaskans do get skin cancer. In every state in the Union a person can acquire tuberculosis,

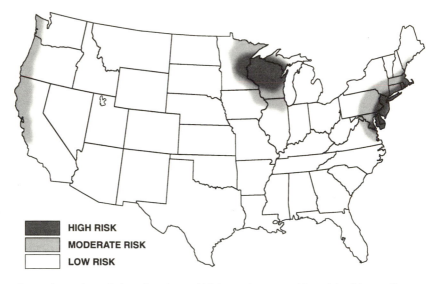

Approximate boundaries of regions of high, moderate, and low risk of Lyme disease in the United States. Within regions marked as high or moderate risks, there are some areas, such as urban areas, in which the risk of Lyme disease is minimal. In general, persons in high-risk areas are about ten times as likely to get infected as those in moderate-risk areas, and one hundred times as likely as those in low-risk areas. In some regions, such as the Rocky Mountains and the desert Southwest, the chances of getting Lyme disease are practically nonexistent. In the southeastern and south-central United States there are areas from which Lyme disease has been reported, but where the transmission of *Borrelia burgdorferi* to people has not been confirmed. *Map by Alan Barbour*

AIDS, gonorrhea, strep throat, dysentery, hepatitis, and influenza. But a person cannot "catch" *B. burgdorferi* in every state. In some places, perhaps most of the land area of the continental United States, it is impossible to become infected, for reasons given in the next chapter.

In North America the annual risk of being infected with *B. burgdorferi* ranges from zero in most of the Rocky Mountain states, such as Wyoming and New Mexico, to about one chance in two hundred for long-term residents of high-risk areas, such as Lyme, Connecticut; Nantucket County, Massachusetts; Hunterdon County, New Jersey; and Westchester County, New York. The highest-risk areas extend along the Atlantic coast from Virginia to Maine. The states with the

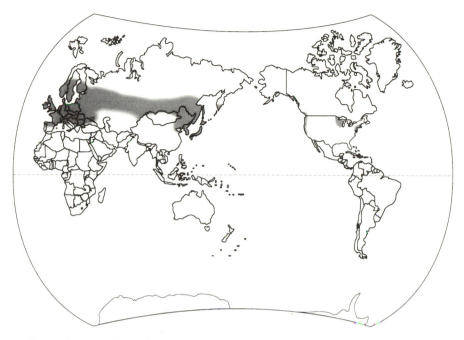

Parts of the world *(shaded areas)* in which Lyme disease definitely is known to occur, or conditions are suitable for its transmission. *Map by Alan Barbour*

highest number of cases per capita are Connecticut, Rhode Island, Delaware, New York, New Jersey, Pennsylvania, Massachusetts, and Maryland. These states account for about 80 percent of the cases reported nationally. To take one state, Connecticut, as an example, the highest rate of Lyme disease is in counties on or near the coast; the lowest incidence is inland, in metropolitan areas.

The incidence of *B. burgdorferi* infection drops perceptibly as one moves farther west, north, and south. An exception is another high-incidence patch of Lyme disease in a region within Minnesota and Wisconsin. The disease also occurs along the West Coast from Southern California to British Columbia, but the frequency on a population basis is only a fraction of what it is in New York and Connecticut. In California, Lyme disease is most common in the northern coastal counties.

Although all states in the United States and all of the provinces of Canada have reported cases of Lyme disease, this does not mean that the disease was acquired in the state. In a state such as Montana or New Mexico, where *B. burgdorferi* has not been found to exist, a case of Lyme disease in a resident is the result of travel to a high-incidence area. Some states such as Georgia and Indiana have a documented presence of *B. burgdorferi* in nature, but the spirochete's presence is sparse enough there that cases of Lyme disease are just as likely to have resulted from travel out of the state as from residence in the state.

One area of North America that confounds public health officials studying Lyme disease is a large inland region that includes several south-central and southeastern states. Physicians in those areas—in particular, parts of Missouri, Arkansas, Oklahoma, Texas, Georgia, and North Carolina—have observed and reported a disease that looks similar to erythema migrans and Lyme disease. The skin rash, like erythema migrans, is associated with a tick bite and seems to respond to antibiotics, yet *B. burgdorferi* has not been proven to be the cause of most of these cases of illness. The ticks most commonly associated with the illness in this region are different from those carrying Lyme disease in the Northeast. One explanation is that there may be another tick-borne agent, perhaps related to *B. burgdorferi*, that can produce an illness with some features similar to Lyme disease.

Lyme disease and *B. burgdorferi* in nature have been documented in almost all countries of western and eastern Europe, from Italy to Finland and from England to Hungary. They occur from the western-most border of Russia to Russia's Pacific coast. In Europe the distribution of Lyme disease cases coincides in part with the distribution of cases of another infectious disease, tick-borne encephalitis. (Encephalitis is an inflammation of the brain.) Regions with a high risk for Lyme disease also generally have a high risk for encephalitis. In central Europe approximately one person in a thousand acquires Lyme disease each year. The rise of reports of Lyme disease during the 1980s in Austria paralleled the increase in reported cases in the United States.

People also get Lyme disease in China, Japan, and Korea. All of the Lyme disease regions of the Old World and the New World have a temperate climate. The infection has not been found in tropical regions such as southeast Asia; in desert areas such as the Sahara; in mountainous regions such as the Rocky Mountains; or in areas where the winters are very harsh, such as regions above the Arctic Circle or at very high altitudes. Lyme disease might occur in Australia, but this has yet to be proven. There is no convincing evidence that the disease infects people living in South America or Africa, although parts of these continents have temperate climates and are home to the types of ticks that might transmit the infection.

In all parts of the world with Lyme disease, the risk of acquiring the disease is highest where there are forested areas containing deer and ticks. But a high-risk area may be as close as one's backyard or a nature reserve just down the street. Many of the riskiest places are in heavily populated suburban areas such as Westchester County, close to New York City; or the suburbs just outside of Munich, Germany, or Vienna, Austria. Associating the risk of Lyme disease exclusively with hiking or hunting in the backwoods or wilderness regions is a misconception. Comparatively few people become infected through recreational activities in remote or otherwise unpopulated areas.

One thing that is certain is that it is difficult to become infected if one stays inside one's house. Of course, a dog, a cat, or a person might carry into the house a tick that might subsequently climb onto a shut-in's skin, but generally a person has to go outside to be bitten by a tick. This may involve as short a distance as a walk across one's lawn or as long a distance as a hike through a forest. Lyme disease ticks, unlike flies, spiders, and cockroaches, have yet to adapt to life inside human habitats. (There are other ticks—for instance, the ones that transmit the disease known as relapsing fever—that reside inside rustic houses and cabins. These ticks occasionally pose indoor threats as vectors of relapsing fever in parts of the western United States and Canada.)

There are two age groups in which Lyme disease is more common: children aged five to fourteen years, and adults aged thirty to forty-nine. This is most likely because of their outdoor exposures around residences. Children and young adolescents play outside, while older adolescents and young adults spend more time in cars and in urban settings, and live in apartments away from forests. People in their thirties and forties are more likely to have started families and to live in the suburbs.

Who Is Tracking and Studying Lyme Disease?

Investigations of Lyme disease and *B. burgdorferi* infection go beyond counting cases and measuring trends and distribution patterns. This work is ongoing, of course, and is primarily carried out by local and state health departments and by the federal agency called the Centers for Disease Control and Prevention (commonly known as the CDC). The main facility for the CDC is located in Atlanta, Georgia, but it's the branch in Fort Collins, Colorado, that focuses on Lyme disease. This may seem odd, since Colorado is a state without documented transmission of the disease to humans; one might suppose that the CDC's Lyme disease facility would be centered at or near the areas with the highest risk of infection. But the Fort Collins facility has for many years focused on other arthropod-borne diseases and for that reason was considered an appropriate place for Lyme disease activities.

In addition to its tracking work on Lyme disease, the CDC provides educational materials to the public (addresses for the CDC and other organizations may be found at the end of this book). Moreover, the CDC carries out research on the disease in its own institutional laboratories and in field studies and provides research grants and contracts to local and state health departments, universities, and foundations. After its admittedly slow beginning in laboratory and field activities, the CDC has taken a leading role in coordinating efforts to improve the reliability of diagnostic tests for Lyme disease and to prevent the infection.

Another federal institution that has long studied Lyme disease is the National Institutes of Health, better known as the NIH. Since 1977 the NIH has supported basic and applied research on Lyme disease. The Montana branch of the NIH is where *B. burgdorferi* was discovered. Some of this research is carried out in NIH facilities, principally at the Rocky Mountain Laboratories. Although the NIH, like the CDC, is part of the federal Public Health Service, its mission is principally basic research and not disease tracking and public education. The term *basic research* has for many people the connotation of "ivory tower" impracticality. "What's the advantage of studying phenomena without having a clear practical application in mind?" they might ask. An example—one of the many that could be selected—of the benefit of basic research is the discovery of the Lyme disease agent itself. As related earlier in this chapter, this discovery was made by scientists carrying out basic research.

Most of the Lyme disease research funded by the NIH is carried out in the laboratories and fieldwork installations of scientists and investigators who are based at other public or private institutions, including universities, medical schools, schools of public health, and other nonprofit research institutes. The NIH also provides some support for small companies in their development of such practical products as diagnostic tests and vaccines for Lyme disease. For all these research programs, there is a highly competitive application process. The applications are evaluated for merit and feasibility by experts drawn from outside of the NIH itself, and applications for work on Lyme disease are evaluated alongside applications for projects on other infections. Overall, no more than about one of the grant applications in five will ever receive funding. There is not enough money in the budget to go around.

There are other United States federal agencies, including the armed services, that also carry out or support research on Lyme disease, but their activities are dwarfed by those of the NIH and the CDC. Some individual states, such as New York, Connecticut, and New Jersey, among others in the high-risk zone, also sponsor research on the disease. But again, the funds for such research are limited, and most of the states' resources for Lyme disease are devoted to providing medical care to patients without insurance; tracking and measuring the infection; assessing the accuracy of reports of Lyme disease; developing educational programs; and controlling ticks. In many financially strapped states, the efforts cannot keep up with the increasing caseload. In Canada, Europe, Russia, and Asia similar tracking, control, and research activities are being carried out by a combination of governmental, educational, and commercial institutions.

Large and small companies are doing research on Lyme disease, principally to develop new diagnostic tests and vaccines. The development costs for a new vaccine for use in humans may be as high as $100 million. In most cases the companies are applying the discoveries made by basic scientists in governmental or university laboratories. For instance, a human vaccine undergoing field trials uses a protein discovered in an NIH lab in Montana and investigated as a vaccine in animals by researchers at universities in Connecticut and Germany.

Some Lyme disease research in the United States is also supported by private nonprofit groups that focus on Lyme disease. The two principal groups supporting this research are the Lyme Disease Foundation, based in Hartford, Connecticut, and the American Lyme Disease Foundation, in Westchester County, New York. Both of these groups develop educational materials for health professionals and for lay people. The Lyme Disease Foundation publishes its own scientific journal on Lyme disease and related disorders. Patients and other interested persons can contact these organizations to receive information about the disease (see Resources, below). These foundations have also organized and presented conferences on Lyme disease. They are active in promoting federal and state support of Lyme disease research and prevention.

At a local level are many patient support groups for people with Lyme disease. These are usually started by one or two individuals in a community and grow by word of mouth and distribution of literature. Some national foundations in the United States refer patients to the Lyme disease support group in their area. There is now a loosely organized network of such groups that share information and newsletters with titles such as *Lyme Disease Update*. Communication occurs by phone, fax, and electronic mail; Lyme disease information and discussions can be found on the Internet. Lyme disease support groups are found in almost every state and Canadian province, even in areas where there is no evidence of transmission of *B. burgdorferi* infection to people.

The support groups provide information about the disease, re-ferrals to physicians, a sympathetic ear to those with frustrating illnesses, and a forum for discussions and the sharing of experiences. Many of the persons participating in the support groups have long-term conditions that they themselves, or physicians or other care-givers, have called chronic Lyme disease. Many of the people in the groups have experienced little or no relief after standard antibiotic therapies for Lyme disease.

There are some disparities between views about Lyme disease ad-vanced by members of the patient support groups and views of the disease fostered by governmental and academic institutions—one of the most contentious areas being how Lyme disease is diagnosed. This is the subject we examine in Chapters 4 and 5. But first we con-sider how *B. burgdorferi* exists in nature and why certain activities put people and their pets at risk of the disease.

An Infection from Nature: The Ecology of Lyme Disease

Lyme disease is an accident by all accounts. Few if any people with the disease would say that getting the infection was their intention or was in any way beneficial to them. And from the microorganism's point of view—if this can be imagined—migration to a human being is a dead end. From its human host there is almost no chance that the Lyme disease agent will be passed on elsewhere. The presence and spread of *Borrelia burgdorferi* in the world depends on other animals, not on people. The fact is that humans are ineffective at transmitting the microorganisms.

Ticks pass the infectious agent from one type of animal to another. Ticks are the transmitters, or *vectors*, of Lyme disease in the sense that mosquitoes are the vectors of malaria and fleas are the vectors of bubonic plague microorganisms. Ticks themselves become infected with the microorganism, but this is not sufficient for *B. burgdorferi* to prosper—to be maintained—in nature. For this to happen there also needs to be a supply, or *reservoir*, of the agent in animals. What happens is that an infected tick bites an animal, which develops the infection; an uninfected tick then bites the infected animal, becomes infected itself, and bites another animal, and so on. People are as poor reservoirs as they are transmitters. Compared to some wild animals and even pet dogs, humans are infrequently infected. If a person does happen to become infected, the chance that another tick will bite him or her and pick up the infection is very small.

When people accidentally become targets for an infectious organism that most often infects animals, this is called a *zoonosis* (pronounced "zoh-oh-noh-sis"). Other zoonoses include Rocky Mountain spotted fever, typhus, brucellosis, plague, rabies, psittacosis ("parrot fever"), cat scratch disease, and trichinosis. Some of these are not familiar names to most people, and the diseases are not very common infections of humans now. Like the hantavirus infections in the southwestern United States, however, they could suddenly increase in numbers. Of all zoonoses in the United States, Lyme disease is at present the most frequent, with the exception of certain types of food poisoning.

Most infections of people are not zoonoses. The majority of infectious diseases that we collectively experience are restricted to humans and, perhaps, related primates. People are the critical reservoirs for infections such as gonorrhea, tuberculosis, herpes, AIDS, "strep throat," hepatitis, and the common cold. Preventing gonorrhea and tuberculosis means stopping the spread of the infection from one person to another. Preventing Lyme disease and many other zoonoses means either removing people from harm's way (that is, the vector's way) or eliminating or reducing the infectious agent in the environment.

Accomplishing either of these goals requires understanding how the Lyme disease agent, *B. burgdorferi*, is maintained in nature and how it is spread to people. This is called the *ecology of Lyme disease*. Ecology is the study of the relationships between organisms—from whale-sized to microscopic—and their environments. For Lyme disease this means taking into account characteristics of the infectious agent, the vectors, and the reservoirs, as well as the landscapes and conditions that foster transmission of the infection. Gaining knowledge about the biology of *B. burgdorferi* and the ecology of Lyme disease means making better-informed choices about lowering one's personal risk for infection.

The Agent
Overview of Disease-Causing Agents

Infections are invasions of our bodies by smaller forms of life. Not all of the microorganisms we carry produce infections, though. In fact, most usually do not. We have microorganisms in our intestines and our mouths and on our skins, but these are usually "fellow travelers," not true infectious agents, because they do not enter our tissues or otherwise cause harm. The mouth and intestine are like donut holes: "inside" the donut in a sense, but still outside the dough, the substance of the donut.

With the exception of some parasitic worms, which are composed of many cells, infectious agents are either viruses or one-celled creatures. In most infections the microorganism penetrates between or into a person's cells. This could be through the respiratory tract, as in tuberculosis or influenza, through the stomach and intestine, as in cholera and dysentery, through the genitals, as in HIV and gonorrhea, or through the skin, as in Lyme disease.

Some do not consider viruses true forms of life because viruses are utterly dependent on the host cells for their duplication. Viruses are essentially well-organized bags of genes and proteins that can manipulate a bacterial, animal, or plant cell's machinery into making more of the same. Viruses cannot eat, respire, or excrete the way that living cells can. Well-known human infections caused by viruses are AIDS, hepatitis, influenza, measles, and common colds.

Single-celled infectious organisms can be fungi, protozoa, or bacteria. Fungi were at one time classified as plants because of their plantlike qualities. Mushrooms, baker's yeast, and bread mold are generally noninfectious fungi. More dangerous for humans are fungi such as *Candida albicans*, the yeast that produces infections of the vagina and throat. Protozoa are generally more animallike than plantlike in structure and behavior. The amebas and paramecia observed in a microscope slide of pond water are protozoa. The infections caused by protozoa include malaria, sleeping sickness, and amebic dysentery.

Lyme disease is caused by a bacterium. Bacteria fundamentally differ from protozoa and fungi in their structure and chemistry. For these and other reasons, they belong in a separate kingdom from other forms of life. Within each kingdom of life are a number of subdivisions; and the subdivision of bacteria that contains the Lyme disease agent is the "spirochetes." Members of the spirochete group are as different from members of another division of bacteria as birds are from clams.

The separate grouping of spirochetes is justified. They are one of the most distinctive forms of bacteria, in their appearance and their behavior. Spirochetes have a spiral or wavy shape (hence their name), and they move through liquids and the tight spaces between cells either as a screw moves through wood or as a snake moves over the ground. The movement is accomplished through the action of a biological motor that rotates or undulates the spirochete. Spirochetes have two membranes—outer and inner—that enclose genes, enzymes, fats, and sugars. Like other bacteria, spirochetes cannot be seen by the unaided eye. A microscope that magnifies at least a hundred times is needed to see most spirochetes. Even then, the spirochete's extremely narrow width requires special optics or stains to make it visible.

Classification of Spirochetes

Just as there are different varieties of mollusks (such as snails, clams, and squids), and just as plants may be subdivided into ferns, pines, and mosses, so the spirochete group may be further subdivided. Spirochete types differ from one another in size, physiology, and the environments they thrive in. Some spirochetes are what is known as "free-living," which means that they can live outside of an animal. They are not as unrestricted as the name implies, however. Their ecological niches may be very limited—for instance, they may exist only at a depth of a meter or so in a mud flat.

But most known spirochetes are not free-living. They exist and propagate only within another living being. Their hosts supply not only nutrition but also safety from climate, microscopic predators, and other hazards of the outside world. Free-living microorganisms have a variety of ways of coping with changing and inhospitable conditions they encounter, whereas more dependent organisms in effect jettison their lifeboats once the harbor of an animal host is reached. They can handle many situations in the "harbor" itself but are poorly equipped for ventures beyond the animal's boundaries. Furthermore, many host-associated spirochetes are so specialized that they are restricted to certain types of animals. One spirochete occupies the intestine of only one species of termite. In contrast, the Lyme disease spirochete is comparatively nondiscriminating in its choice of hosts.

Some of these host-associated spirochetes, including *B. burgdorferi*, can be grown in the laboratory outside of an animal, but special conditions are required. For example, the culture medium for growing Lyme disease spirochetes contains about fifty different ingredients, including complex mixtures of proteins, fats, and vitamins. Most host-associated spirochetes have never been propagated outside of an animal, because scientists have not identified all of their particular needs.

The Lyme disease agents belong to a *genus* called *Borrelia* within the group of spirochetes. This genus contains other species besides *B. burgdorferi*. All species of *Borrelia* have in common the need for both an arthropod vector and a mammalian or bird reservoir. Before the discovery of the cause of Lyme disease, *Borrelia* species were primarily known as the agents of relapsing fever and an infection of poultry. One form of relapsing fever is transmitted by certain types of ticks and is indigenous to Eurasia and the Americas. In North America the tick-borne forms of relapsing fever occur in western and some southern states in the United States, the western provinces of Canada, and northern Mexico. In the United States, fewer than one hundred cases of relapsing fever are reported in most years. Because the relapsing fever *Borrelia* species and *B. burgdorferi* are closely related, sometimes the diseases are confused with one another on the basis of the blood test for Lyme disease. Several ill people in west Texas were mistakenly thought on the basis of blood tests to have Lyme disease when relapsing fever was the actual cause of their illnesses.

The second major form of relapsing fever *Borrelia* has only been found in humans and is passed by body lice, which are insects, and not by ticks. The louse-borne form of relapsing fever is at present limited in its distribution to parts of northern and central Africa. In past decades, though, louse-borne relapsing fever has caused millions of cases of disease in people, including many in the United States and Europe. The most recent widespread epidemic of this fever was during and just after World War II in the Middle East and North Africa. As with plague, an outbreak of louse-borne relapsing fever can quickly grow from inconsequential to epidemic proportions.

Another type of spirochete causes syphilis and is in a different genus from the *Borrelia*. The syphilis agent, *Treponema pallidum*, infects only human beings and has not been cultivated in the laboratory. Syphilis is spread from person to person by sexual and other forms of intimate physical contact. There is no arthropod or any other nonhuman vector of syphilis. The spirochetes that cause syphilis, relapsing fever, and Lyme disease have in common the ability to penetrate into the brains of animals and, in some cases, to remain there for extended periods, causing temporary or permanent brain damage. One of the most feared results of syphilis in the days before penicillin was infection of the brain, and many patients with chronic syphilis of the brain populated the mental hospitals of the eighteenth and nineteenth centuries.

The Vector
How Ticks Are Classified

A tick bite hurts less than a bee sting. Indeed, most tick bites are not even felt by the person who is being bitten. And ticks themselves are not as irritating as the mosquitoes or biting flies that swarm around one's head. Yet for most people ticks seem to be more repulsive and chilling than other blood-sucking or stinging arthropods. Ticks are in the same disgust league as leeches and tapeworms.

For all the blood they take, mosquitoes spend little time on a person's body; they fill up within minutes through their tube-like mouth and move on. Most ticks, in contrast, are more leisurely feeders, preferring a long meal with their heads burrowed into the skin. It's very unpleasant to discover a partially embedded tick, purplish and swollen with blood, on one's own body or the body of a loved one. Fastened tight like that, a tick cannot simply be brushed away like a gnat or a flea. Removing the creature takes skill and patience, if the mouth and head are not to be left behind in the skin. Finding a tick crawling on clothes or skin is better than finding it after it has become embedded; on the other hand, finding one tick means that another one may have escaped detection and settled in elsewhere on the body for a feed.

But ticks are more than creepy nuisances. They are ideally suited for passing on infectious microorganisms. Bacteria, viruses, and parasites that populate the blood of their hosts may be carried from one host to another by a tick. The tick that parasitizes people and other animals is itself taken advantage of by its smaller passengers. Because the interval between feedings for a tick is measured in months and even years, a microorganism that goes along for the ride in the tick until reaching its next vertebrate host has to be adapted for life in the very different environment within the tick. Some tick-borne infectious agents spend more time in the arthropod than they do in a mammal or bird.

Ticks are members of the phylum Arthropoda, the most diverse and populous group of animals on earth. The arthropods include arachnids, insects, centipedes, millipedes, and crustacea, such as lobsters and crabs. Like other arthropods, ticks have their skeletons or supporting hard body parts on the outside instead of inside. Most arthropods have a body divided into separate segments. Their internal temperatures change as the temperature of the environment changes, instead of remaining at the even, warm temperature of mammals and birds. Arthropods do not have true blood or blood vessels. Instead, their organs are bathed directly in a liquid carrying oxygen and nutrients. Arthropods cannot make antibodies; they do not have lymphocytes, the adaptable and protective cells of our own immune systems. Instead, they contend with infectious agents with a few preformed chemicals and cells that serve as scavengers. Compared with a vertebrate's immune system, an arthropod's is very primitive.

Among arthropods, ticks are in the group Arachnida, which also includes spiders, scorpions, and mites. Ticks and mites are closely related and form a group, Acarina, separate from other arachnids. Tiny mites are common, harmless residents of people's eyelash and hair follicles. Other mites cause the skin disease scabies. Many types of mites are free-living and can be found in the soil, on plants, and in and around the home. Some people develop respiratory allergies, such as hay fever and asthma, to the feces and skeletons of mites living in our houses.

Adult arachnids have eight legs or appendages instead of the six characteristic of insects. Ticks and mites differ from other arachnids in having an unsegmented body. Arachnids have simple eyes and tactile body hairs to feel their environment. Some can sense the presence in the air of certain chemicals, such as carbon dioxide, and this ability guides them to an animal breathing out this gas. Most arachnids are carnivorous but free-living; they actively capture their food, which is usually smaller in size. Ticks, on the other hand, are parasites; they feed off a larger animal.

Like vampire bats, ticks take their sustenance primarily from blood. Parts of the tick's mouth are adapted for piercing and sucking; its teeth are turned backwards to hold fast in the skin, for example. Generally a tick's meals are far apart—separated by months or years—so it must make good use of its opportunities. For a tick to obtain a year's worth of blood, it must remain unnoticed for several hours to days. The bite provokes no pain, and the saliva that the tick injects into the skin prevents the clotting of blood and inflammation of the surrounding area. If the buried head and mouth of the tick were to produce itching and pain, the person's attention would be drawn to the feeding tick—leading to its removal.

The tick's structure allows its abdomen to swell with blood to many times its usual size. In this bloated state ticks are more easily noticed on the body, but by then it may be too late to stop the infection. Once the blood enters the tick's intestine, it is slowly absorbed into cells lining the gut, where it is broken down to its constituent proteins, carbohydrates, nucleic acids, and fats, the simple chemicals that the tick's own cells can use.

If the tick feeds on an animal infected with *B. burgdorferi*, some spirochetes may enter the tick's intestine along with the blood meal. They will survive and may proliferate inside the tick's gut, an environment hospitable to them. The inside of a mosquito or biting fly is not conducive to spirochetes' survival and growth because, unlike ticks, mosquitoes and flies digest blood inside the intestine itself instead of within the cells in the lining of the intestine. The chemicals and enzymes that break down the blood in the mosquito's intestine also kill the spirochetes. This is one reason that mosquitoes and biting flies are poor transmitters of Lyme disease.

In ticks, many of the spirochetes remain in the safe environment of the intestine. From there they may be regurgitated up into the site of the bite the next time that the tick feeds. Other spirochetes pass through the intestinal cell layer into the body cavity itself. From there they may migrate to the tick's salivary glands. These glands, on either side of the mouth parts in the head, may be another source of infection when the tick consumes blood and skin tissue fluid.

One advantage in the battle against infection is the lag period between the time when a tick begins to feed and the time at which infectious spirochetes pass from tick to the animal. In some experiments it has taken at least one day, sometimes two, for the spirochetes to become active enough to produce an infection. The entry of blood into the feeding tick stimulates the spirochete to leave the intestine and journey to the tick's salivary glands. A proposed reason for the one- to two-day delay in transmission of infection is that it is necessary for the spirochetes to first move to the salivary glands. The practical advantage of this phenomenon may be that if a tick is removed within the first day or two after it has embedded, the chances of infection are lower than if the tick had been feeding for longer.

Like other types of arthropods, some ticks go through different stages between hatching from an egg and achieving adulthood. Growth occurs by metamorphosis, called *molting*. As the tick passes through the various stages between molts, its appearance changes. The earlier forms are not just smaller versions of the adult. The earliest stage after hatching is the *larva*. The larval tick has three pairs of legs instead of the four pairs of later stages. Once a larval tick has a blood meal, it molts to the next stage, the *nymph*. The nymph is bigger than a larva and has its own unique features. For a nymph to change into an adult, the final stage, it also must have a blood meal. The adult female must feed if it is to have the energy and body mass necessary to produce eggs. For many types of ticks the interval between the different stages is usually a year, sometimes two years. A larva may change to a nymph after its meal in the spring, summer, or fall. The nymphal form of that tick has to survive the winter before it feeds.

Lyme Disease Ticks

It is as simple as this: no ticks, no Lyme disease. But only a few types of ticks are capable of spreading this infection. We need not

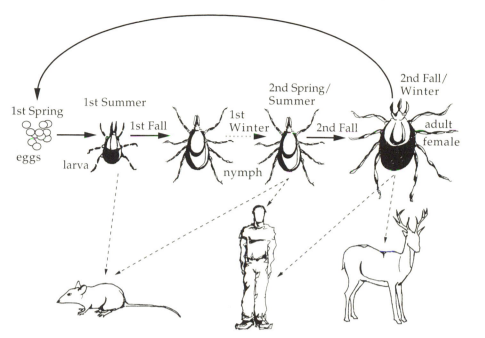

Two-year life cycle of *Ixodes scapularis* in the northern United States. There are four life or developmental stages for hard-bodied ticks such as *I. scapularis*: egg, larva, nymph, and adult. Transitions between stages are indicated by *solid arrows* in the picture; the usual period of the year during which each change occurs is given above the arrow. The cycle for an individual tick begins in the spring of the first year. Then an adult female tick who had fed on a deer during the fall or winter lays her eggs. The larva emerges from the eggs in the spring or summer and feeds on a mouse, and may become infected with *Borrelia burgdorferi* from the mouse. (Feeding is indicated by *dashed lines with arrows*.) After feeding, the larva changes to the next stage, a nymph, during the fall. The nymph does not usually feed until it has passed through the first winter *(dotted line and arrow)*. In the spring or summer of the second year the nymph feeds on a small mammal or bird or sometimes a human. Because of the small size of a nymph, people often are not aware of its bite. After its blood meal, the nymph changes to an adult in the late summer or fall. Only about 10 percent of the nymphs make it to the adult stage. The adult female feeds during the fall, winter, and sometimes the early spring on deer and occasionally on other large mammals and humans. During feeding, the adult female mates with a male, who does not feed during this stage. The female produces eggs and then dies. The two-year cycle begins again with the eggs. *Drawing by Nathan Barbour and Alan Barbour*

worry about all ticks, at least with regard to Lyme disease. Other ticks, with genus names such as *Dermacentor* and *Ornithodorus*, bring their own perils, including Rocky Mountain spotted fever, relapsing fever, Colorado tick fever, ehrlichiosis, and tularemia. With the exceptions of *Dermacentor variabilis*, a vector of Rocky Mountain spotted fever, and *Amblyomma americanum*, a possible vector of ehrlichiosis, these other disease-carrying ticks do not occur in the areas that have the highest risks for Lyme disease. Relapsing fever and Colorado tick fever usually occur in regions of western North America that have few if any cases of Lyme disease.

In Europe earlier in this century, the skin rash erythema migrans was observed to follow the bite of a particular type of tick, one common name of which was the "sheep tick." The full genus-and-species name of this tick is *Ixodes ricinus*. (Following the pattern seen above, and also used below for other Latin names, it is abbreviated as *I. ricinus*.) In the 1970s, medical detective work implicated a related tick, *Ixodes scapularis*, as the vector of Lyme disease in the northeastern and north-central United States. *I. scapularis* is often called the "deer tick" in the Northeast because it is found so frequently on deer. (The northern form of *I. scapularis* has also been called *"Ixodes dammini."*) *I. scapularis* is found in the southeast and south-central states, as well. The southern form of *I. scapularis* has had the common name "black-legged tick." The southern form of the species poses less of a threat than the northern form. Fewer of the southern ticks are infected with *B. burgdorferi,* and the southern ticks are less apt to frequent places where humans tread. They also prefer to feed on other animal hosts. Humans are more commonly bitten by adults than by nymphs of the southern form of *I. scapularis.*

Ixodes pacificus (the western black-legged tick) in the western United States and Canada and *Ixodes persulcatus* in Russia and Asia are the known vectors of *B. burgdorferi* infection elsewhere. The Lyme disease agent has been found in *Ixodes uriae* ticks infesting sea birds near the Arctic and Antarctic Circles and in *Ixodes spinipalpis* ticks in Colorado near the Rocky Mountains. The latter two ticks are not associated with Lyme disease, because they rarely if ever feed on humans.

The ticks that transmit Lyme disease live about two years. *I. scapularis* larvae, which are not much larger than the period at the end of this sentence, hatch in the summer from eggs laid by the adult female that spring. They generally feed on a field mouse or other rodent host that summer or early fall. The larvae change to nymphs the first year; these nymphs pass through that winter without feeding. The following spring and summer the nymphs feed on a rodent or other small animal. At least three out of four Lyme disease cases in the northeastern and north-central United States are from the bite of a nymphal tick that occurs sometime between May and August. Most of the bites are unnoticed because the nymphs are so small—about the size of a poppy seed.

In the second year, the nymph changes to an adult after feeding. The larger adult ticks, especially the females, are more likely to be noticed by people. *I. scapularis* adults bite deer and other large mammals, such as humans. The adults feed later in the year than nymphs and larvae and may remain active even as temperatures drop to just above freezing in the late fall. People who develop symptoms of acute Lyme disease infection in the fall in the northeastern and north-central United States have usually been bitten by an adult female tick. In warmer regions of the United States the tick-bite season begins earlier in the spring and lasts until or into winter.

The entire life cycle for *I. scapularis*—from emergence from the egg and progression through larval and nymphal stages, to the laying of eggs by the female—takes two years. In Europe and Russia the cycle for *I. ricinus* may be three years because all stages—not just nymphs—can pass through the winter.

Spirochetes have occasionally been found in other tick species in North America, including *Dermacentor variabilis,* the "dog tick," and *Amblyomma americanum.* The latter, commonly known as the "Lone Star tick" because of a distinctive white spot on the female's back, is a frequent biter of humans in the eastern and south-central United States. Although these tick species can acquire *B. burgdorferi* during feeding, they have not been able to transmit these spirochetes to other hosts in experimental studies. This is a paradoxical finding, because the Lone Star tick has been implicated as the vector of a Lyme disease–

like disorder in Missouri, Georgia, Texas, and other regions of the south-central and southeastern United States. Spirochetes have been identified inside Lone Star ticks, but they are not *B. burgdorferi;* they are another species of *Borrelia.*

Ixodes ticks carry other infections besides Lyme disease. Among them are *babesiosis, tick-borne encephalitis,* and *ehrlichiosis.* Babesiosis is a parasitic disease similar in some features to malaria. The *Babesia microti* parasites infect the blood cells of animals. Humans rarely become sick from an infection. Those who have developed illness from babesiosis have been elderly, have had a serious underlying medical condition, or have been lacking a spleen (an organ that effectively filters infections from the blood). Babesiosis occurs in some of the same locales as Lyme disease in North America and Europe. Some people have had Lyme disease and babesiosis at the same time. These people generally have been sicker than those with Lyme disease alone. In some cases of mixed infections, symptoms of babesiosis persisted after appropriate treatment for Lyme disease had been completed.

Tick-borne encephalitis, or TBE, occurs in Europe and Russia but not North America. The disease is caused by a virus, not a bacterium like *B. burgdorferi* or a parasite like *Babesia microti.* The virus invades the central nervous system—thus the term *encephalitis,* which means inflammation of the brain. The result of a TBE infection may be as benign as a fever and headache or severe enough to produce confusion, body weakness, or even coma. For several years there has been a vaccine available in Europe for the prevention of TBE.

Ehrlichiosis is another zoonotic infection in North America that is increasing in incidence. In some areas ehrlichiosis is more common than Rocky Mountain spotted fever. The disease is caused by a bacterium that can only live inside of cells. In its early stages ehrlichiosis may be confused with Lyme disease; the symptoms are fever, headache, and muscle aches all over. There have been several deaths from the disease. A laboratory test tip-off for ehrlichiosis is a lower-than-normal white blood cell count. One form of ehrlichiosis appears to be transmitted by *I. scapularis* ticks in the north-central and northeastern United States. Another form has been associated with *Am-*

blyomma americanum in the south-central and southeastern parts of the country. Some patients have Lyme disease and ehrlichiosis at the same time.

Reservoirs

Ticks can be a dead end for Lyme disease bacteria. The spirochetes remain alive and may even multiply inside the tick's body, but they seldom are passed from a female tick to its offspring. For the spirochetes to spread in nature, for their numbers to increase, the infected tick must feed on another animal, thereby passing on the organism through that animal to other ticks—and on and on—to enlarge the population.

Many types of mammals and birds are capable not only of being infected with *B. burgdorferi* but also of passing the microorganisms on to another tick, thus completing a vector-reservoir-vector cycle. Larvae, the toddlers of tick development, feed for about four days on their first meals. About 99 percent of the larvae of *I. scapularis* are free of spirochetes even if their adult mothers and fathers had been infected. The larvae acquire the bacteria by feeding on an infected host. In the case of deer ticks this is usually a wild field mouse, called *Peromyscus leucopus* for its white feet (*leucos* is Greek for "white"). This type of mouse is numerous in rural and suburban areas of central and eastern North America. In some regions more than half the mice are infected with Lyme disease bacteria, and in these mice the infection persists for months, providing a continuous reservoir of the spirochetes for many ticks. In high-risk areas for Lyme disease the chances that a larva will become infected is at least one in four.

Other reservoirs of *B. burgdorferi* besides white-footed mice contribute to infection of ticks. Unlike many other ticks, which are limited in the types of animals they successfully feed from, *I. scapularis* can parasitize a variety of animals, including birds, such as robins, and other small- and medium-sized mammals, such as raccoons, squirrels, and voles. Thus, eliminating or controlling infections in the field mice would not necessarily solve the problem. These animals are also the hosts for nymphs, when they feed. If a population of ticks had about a 25-percent rate of infection with *B. burgdorferi* at the nymphal stage, its infection rate might top 50 percent after the nymphs fed and became adults. The chance of infection doubles with each meal. The nymphs generally feed before the larvae feed, thereby increasing the chances that a larva will pick an infected animal for its blood meal.

The prevalence of *B. burgdorferi* infection in ticks differs between geographic areas. Even within the northeastern United States—the hotbed of Lyme disease in North America—tick infection rates vary from less than 1 percent in some regions to more than 70 percent in others. The percentage of ticks that are infected in a given region is a good predictor of the frequency of Lyme disease there. Information about the prevalence of *Ixodes* ticks and the prevalence of Lyme disease bacteria in the ticks in a given area can be obtained from the local health department. Another source of information is the entomology department of a nearby university. (Entomology is the study of insects and arachnids.)

In comparison to the northeastern and some north-central states, the southern and western United States have a lower prevalence of infected ticks and, consequently, a low frequency of Lyme disease. One of the reasons for these lower rates of infection is the feeding preferences of the larval and nymphal ticks. In the southern United States immature *I. scapularis* ticks feed primarily upon lizards. Lyme disease spirochetes cannot infect reptiles, and thus, lizards cannot be reservoirs of infection. Only about 1 to 5 percent of nymphs and adults of the southern form of *I. scapularis* are infected with *B. burgdorferi*.

Spirochete infection rates are also in the 1 to 5 percent range in *I. pacificus* in the western United States and Canada. Immature *I. pacificus* ticks usually feed on lizards and not mammals. The Lyme disease agent is maintained in nature in California and other locations inhabited by *I. pacificus* through another transmission cycle. A different but related tick, *Ixodes neotomae,* which only rarely bites humans, is the vector for Lyme disease bacteria, and a wood rat is the reservoir in this second cycle. *I. pacificus* might occasionally acquire the spirochetes when it feeds on an infected wood rat or other small mammal instead of its usual lizard host. The infrequency of this event accounts for the infrequency of the spirochetes in western ticks. With its lower rate of tick infections, the West Coast region of the United States has overall a risk of Lyme disease only one-tenth to one-hundredth as great as the risk in the Northeast. Although *B. burgdorferi* has been identified in *I. spinipalpis* ticks in Colorado, there are no instances of transmission to humans in that state. *I. spinipalpis* much prefers wood rats to people for a meal.

I. ricinus in Europe and *I. persulcatus* in the former Soviet Union and Asia have ecologies that are similar to that of the deer tick in North America. Immature ticks of the Old World species feed primarily upon mammals and birds instead of reptiles. Consequently, spirochete infection rates in parts of Europe and Russia are as high as those found in the northeastern United States. Reservoirs for Lyme disease agents in Eurasia include voles and rabbits as well as local varieties of field mice. Some adult Old World ticks feed on sheep and cattle as well as deer.

In Europe and Asia there are additional transmission cycles, producing an ecology that is more complex than that in the northeastern United States. In these other cycles the ticks involved seldom if ever bite people, but they serve to maintain the spirochetes in nature. In Switzerland, *B. burgdorferi* is in hedgehogs and the ticks that infest them. In northern Sweden, as well as some other locations near the Arctic and Antarctic Circles, the Lyme disease agent is in ticks that only feed on seabirds, such as gulls and albatrosses. The ticks that carry Lyme disease in Japan and China primarily parasitize domestic animals and people. Infected cows and other domestic animals may be the primary reservoir of the infection in these countries, or there may be additional cycles that are the underlying source of the spirochetes. In Australia a tick-associated disease similar to Lyme disease has been described, but the agent has not yet been identified in ticks, wildlife, or people.

Explanations for the Rise in Lyme Disease

Lyme disease and erythema migrans were noted in North America several decades after they were first reported in Europe. This difference in timetable cannot be attributed to the rash being overlooked by U.S. physicians, since the skin rash of early *B. burgdorferi* infection is distinctive enough that they would not have missed it. In fact, the first medical article about erythema migrans in U.S. citizens reported only on people who had acquired the disease while they visited or lived in Europe. The first known case of Lyme disease acquired in the United States was in 1962. These facts lead to this question: is Lyme disease a recent importation to North America from Europe or elsewhere in the Old World? Soon after the discovery of *B. burgdorferi* it was suspected that the migration of Lyme disease from Europe across the Atlantic took place in the twentieth century. But more recent findings suggest otherwise.

What initially suggested a recent importation was the similarity between different isolates of *B. burgdorferi* in the United States, a finding that contrasted with the greater diversity of Lyme disease spirochetes in Europe. If *B. burgdorferi* had been in North America for a long time, it would be expected to appear in a variety of forms, too. There was a problem with the recent-importation theory, though: how could the appearance of Lyme disease at the same time in places as far apart as Connecticut, Minnesota, and California be accounted for? Although *Ixodes* ticks can be carried by birds from one place to another, ticks generally move from one place to another or expand their range slowly. Providing further doubt about the recent-importation theory was the discovery of strains of *B. burgdorferi* in California and southeastern states which differed from anything found in the eastern United States.

The evidence now indicates that *B. burgdorferi* was in North America before Europeans first stepped on that continent's shores. The microorganisms may be "new" to North America by a geologic or evolutionary yardstick, which measures millions of years. But the major migration would still have taken place several thousands of years ago, at the time of the land bridge between Eurasia and North America, not a few decades ago, during the era of steamship travel from Marseilles and New York. From descriptions of colonial forests and of ticks by explorers and the first settlers, it is apparent that conditions for *B. burgdorferi* transmission were present in North America hundreds of years ago. A description of a tick collected in New York in 1749 is consistent with *I. scapularis*.

The mildness of the symptoms of acute Lyme disease in comparison to those of infections such as smallpox, cholera, tuberculosis, and typhus, which affected many North Americans through the nineteenth century, may have allowed Lyme disease to escape public notice. But that does not explain the continuing obscurity of the disease in North America for the first three-quarters of the twentieth century. Those more deadly infectious diseases were already in decline by 1900, and as stated, physicians probably did not overlook the hallmark skin rash, erythema migrans. The inescapable conclusion is that Lyme disease is much more frequent now than it was in the first half of the twentieth century. *B. burgdorferi* has reemerged in the environment. Ecological changes in the northeastern and midwestern United States account for the rise of Lyme disease as an individual threat and a public health problem.

Here falls into place—after the agent, the vector, and the reservoir—the fourth piece of the ecological puzzle of North American Lyme disease: deer. These large mammals can be infected with *B. burgdorferi,* but deer are not the principal reservoirs for the infection. Their importance for the ecology of Lyme disease instead derives from their contributions to the survival of the *Ixodes* ticks. In North America the white-tailed deer (*Odocoileus virginianus*) is the critical host for the maintenance of *I. scapularis* populations in nature. Deer are the host of choice for adult ticks. If a female adult tick does not have a blood meal during the summer or fall, it will not be able to produce eggs the next spring. If there are no deer in an area, the numbers of *I. scapularis* ticks will decline over time.

At a time like the present, when deer seem as common as squirrels in some suburbs, it is difficult to conceive of a time when deer were nearly eliminated from the northeastern and midwestern United States. This drastic reduction of the number of deer was the consequence of hunting and deforestation during the seventeenth, eighteenth, and nineteenth centuries. Forests were cleared for homesteads and agriculture and later for industry. Around 1900 there were fewer than two hundred deer in New Jersey, and the sighting of deer tracks made newspaper headlines in communities in Massachusetts and Vermont. In Indiana, white-tailed deer disappeared entirely and were only reintroduced to the state in the 1930s. In Europe deforestation happened over a longer period of time and with generally greater respect for the husbandry of wildlife, but there, too, it had progressed to the point that outside of mountainous regions deer were limited to small areas of woodlands.

In the northeastern United States, there were a few places where deer survived. In a few isolated areas, such as Naushon Island, Massachusetts, deer herds remained. Examination of arthropod collections in museums revealed that *I. scapularis* was present on Long Island at least fifty years ago. Adapting a procedure for matching suspects to crimes—a procedure that was used fancifully for recreating dinosaurs in the film *Jurassic Park*—scientists found evidence of the DNA of *B. burgdorferi* in these museum specimens of ticks.

After declining through the nineteenth century and the early part of the twentieth, forested lands made a comeback beginning in the mid-twentieth century. The center of gravity for agricultural activity in the United States moved westward. Eastern farms were abandoned or sold for residences, whose owners preferred trees and woodlands to expanses of grass. The landscape of the northeastern United States changed from one of open fields to deciduous forests. And as the forests returned, so did the deer. Because of "green belts" that extend from outlying forests into cities, deer are now found near the centers of such heavily populated areas as Philadelphia, Pennsylvania; and Berlin, Germany. Other factors resulting in the resurgence of deer were stricter hunting regulations and the decline of the deer's natural predators. If at the turn of the century there were an estimated half a million deer left in the entire United States, by 1990 there were twenty-five million. In some areas there are as many as one hundred deer per square mile.

The mainland invasion by *I. scapularis* from its island refuges was the start of the reappearance of Lyme disease in the northeastern United States. *I. scapularis* made other mainland invasions from offshore islands of New Jersey, New York, and Massachusetts. The tick population of Westchester County, just outside of New York City, has steadily increased over the last several years; in 1985 there were an estimated fourteen thousand victims of bites by *I. scapularis* in

that single county. There was an independent expansion of a population of *I. scapularis* ticks in the north-central United States; these
ticks had been first noted in Wisconsin in 1970. Another possible
launching pad for the reemergence of *B. burgdorferi* in North America was the southeastern United States. In that region *B. burgdorferi*
appears to have been long-established, and there was less deforestation.

In many of these and other regions *I. scapularis* continues to extend its range. From the coastal areas the ticks are moving inland—
for instance, up the Hudson River Valley and the Connecticut River
Valley, and from Cape Cod westward, farther into Massachusetts.
The ticks are now found at northern latitudes at which they had not
previously been seen in human memory in the United States. Lyme
disease now is reported in New Hampshire and Maine. This ex-
tension is in part attributable to reforestation and increase in deer
populations. Migration or other movements of birds carrying the
infection themselves or in their parasite ticks may be another factor.
In Sweden the Lyme disease vector ticks have been found on offshore
islands near the Arctic Circle, where these ticks had not been observed previously. The northward creep of some *Ixodes* species in
the world also indicates that more ticks are surviving the winters at
higher latitudes.

In the western and southeastern United States, the clearing of the
native forests and the killing of deer were less drastic than east of the
Rocky Mountains. The representation of *B. burgdorferi* in California
and in the Southeast may be about the same as it has been for hundreds of years. If the number of infected ticks has not increased over
the last century, however, the human population has. There are millions of people at risk. In the far western and the southeastern United
States many new homes are built close to wilderness or forested areas,
bringing more people into day-to-day contact with the vector and
reservoirs of Lyme disease.

The association between the increase in tick populations and the
increase in Lyme disease has been documented. Less certain is the
role of evolution of the spirochete itself in the emergence of this infection. Could there have been a genetic change, a mutation, in a *Bor-*

relia spirochete which made it more infectious for people and animals? A mutant organism carries a change in its DNA such that one or more of its proteins is different from those of the organism that directly preceded it—in effect, its parent. An example is the albino mutant. Animals with this mutation have an abnormality in one protein which results in a lack of pigmentation in their skin and fur.

Another, more pertinent example is HIV infection and AIDS. It is generally thought that this disease is due to a virus—once restricted to another animal or animals, even up to a few decades ago—that changed or "mutated" to the extent that it could now successfully infect humans and, more important, could be spread from one person to another without recourse to another vector. The HIV virus is related to viruses that infect other primates; probably one of these other primate viruses went through a few or several mutations to become what is now known as HIV.

A comparably recent change in a spirochete may have occurred, too, but it need not have. As stated earlier in this chapter, humans contribute little to the spread of *B. burgdorferi* in nature. Person-to-person spread of Lyme disease does not occur. By contrast, humans are the principal hosts, reservoirs, and vectors of the HIV virus. The AIDS epidemic was possible because a virus changed in a way that was to the virus's advantage. No such fundamental change was required for Lyme disease in humans. *B. burgdorferi*, in comparison to other spirochetes, such as the one that causes syphilis, is less finicky about what kinds of animals it will infect. The Lyme disease agent can proliferate in many types of mammals and birds. If there was a change in a spirochete, it likely occurred thousands or millions of years ago. At that time the hypothetical ancestral spirochete broke out of a tight, restricted relationship with one or a few types of animals and became, to our hazard, more tolerant about who it would live in.

Landscapes and Lyme Disease Risk

Ask any person on the street where someone might pick up a tick, and the answer would likely be "in the forest," "in a wilderness region," "on a hike," or "on a hunting trip." Ticks are usually thought of as hazards only for people away from home or in remote places. They are not generally considered to be domestic threats or nuisances. Although many people do acquire their B. *burgdorferi* infections at a distance from home—perhaps hiking, camping, fishing, or hunting—most cases of Lyme disease in the United States begin with an encounter with a tick living around or close to human residences. The occurrence of Lyme disease in suburban areas has reacquainted communities with the dangers of nature that is close at hand. Residents of some of the most desirable residential areas of the northeastern United States have come to fear spending time in their yards, school grounds, and nature preserves. Other people—less at risk perhaps in the vicinity of their own homes—have chosen to forgo trips and excursions to forests, state and national parks, and wilderness areas because of the fear of Lyme disease.

Apartment dwellers in Manhattan, Moscow, Minneapolis, Zurich, San Francisco, or Stockholm need not be concerned about getting Lyme disease in their urban neighborhoods. The danger instead may come through a job or through recreational activities, if that job or recreation is outdoors and outside the city center. (Green belts extending into the city may bring the danger of Lyme disease into the city, however, and may be considered an exception to the above.) Forestry workers in the Netherlands and England have a five times higher risk of getting B. *burgdorferi* infection than others living in the same areas. Soldiers in Austrian woods and hikers in Swiss mountain areas have about a one-in-ten chance of becoming infected over the course of a summer outdoors. In Sweden, people with weekend and summer homes in an area outside of Stockholm were two to three times more likely to have had B. *burgdorferi* infections than were those who tended to stay in the city. Investigations of Lyme disease cases in California revealed that the risk of disease went up with the number of hours spent hiking on trails and pursuing other outdoor recreations. On Fire Island, New York, one of every hundred seasonal residents became infected one summer; cumulatively, about 10 percent of the summer residents there have had the disease.

Tick vectors of Lyme disease are most likely to be found in densely wooded areas with ground cover and leaves. Woodland paths are used by deer as well as humans, and these may have an especially high number of ticks in the adjacent grass and bushes. Less likely to have ticks are meadows and abandoned fields long overgrown with woody shrubs. The outdoor areas with the lowest risk are farm lands, athletic fields, and beaches, but often these are adjacent to wooded areas. The fairways of the country club may be safe, but there is greater danger than a high score from a ball hooked into the deep rough or the adjoining woods.

Residing close to forests or wood lots provides the greatest domestic threat of Lyme disease. In a Massachusetts town the odds of becoming infected at or near home were directly related to the distance between the home and a forested nature preserve. In California and New York the risk of Lyme disease was higher for people with deer living near their houses. A field study in suburban Westchester County showed that while most ticks were in wood lots and in unmaintained edges between forest and lawn, there were also ticks on ornamental plants and in the lawns of people's homes. Two-thirds of all the lawns with Lyme disease tick vectors in the study had adjoining wood lots. A study in New Jersey showed that in comparison to their disease-free neighbors, children with Lyme disease were more likely to play in their back yard than inside the house or in the front yard. Front yards generally have well-trimmed grass; back yards more often abut a stand of trees or dense shrubs.

Tick Tracking

According to Webster's dictionary, *surveillance* means "watch or observation kept over a person, especially one under suspicion." The military use of the word brings to mind outposts, sentinels, and advance guards. Surveillance of diseases can be similar to this. The watch or observation can be of any known threat in the community. Are Lyme disease cases increasing or decreasing in frequency? What proportion of ticks have *B. burgdorferi* in them? If the number of infected ticks in an area is changing, this will have an impact on disease control efforts and the interpretation of the effectiveness of preventive measures.

Surveillance of Lyme disease also includes a figurative outpost, in the form of an area with little or no local acquisition of the infection at present. This is especially important in areas adjoining those with high or moderate disease risk. The establishment of Lyme disease transmission in new areas can be unpredictable. The ultimate limits to the geographic spread of the disease are unknown at present.

One practical benefit of surveillance—of keeping tabs on the disease's whereabouts—is that it assists in the diagnostic process by providing a reasonably accurate answer for use by the physician who asks, "What is the likelihood that the patient before me has Lyme disease?" As with other zoonotic and vector-transmitted infections, a story of exposure to an environment in which infection transmission occurs is a very important clue for assessing the odds of a person's having the disease. In the past, distributions of reported cases of Lyme disease in the United States have not coincided with the distribution of infected ticks, and as the following chapters describe, many of the suspected cases of Lyme disease in areas without infected ticks were not actually *B. burgdorferi* infection. Only a few cases in these areas could be accounted for by true Lyme disease that was acquired by travel to an acknowledged high-risk area. If there was wider appreciation by a community's physicians and its residents that Lyme disease transmission in their area was either an impossibility or extremely unlikely, the number of misdiagnoses would decline. We might consider that, similarly, the diagnosis of malaria is seldom made in North Dakota, because physicians and public health workers there recognize that there is no transmission of that tropical parasite in that state or the adjoining ones.

Surveillance entails recording and confirming cases reported to be Lyme disease, but this infection in humans represents only a tip of the *B. burgdorferi* iceberg. Detecting the spirochete in ticks or rodent reservoirs is an effective way to assess the infection's presence, the risk to residents and visitors, and trends for the future. *B. burgdorferi* infections are a hundredfold or so more common in the ticks and field mice of a community than in its citizens, and advances in biotechnology allow measurements to be made of the spirochete in samples taken from animals, avoiding the need to grow the fastidious organism in the laboratory. Trapped rodents can be tested and then released; the animals do not need to be killed.

In spite of its citizens' and media's interest in Lyme disease, the United States is behind other countries in knowing where its disease vectors are, and in what numbers. The distribution of *I. ricinus* and *I. persulcatus* ticks in Europe and Russia has been known for two decades. Methods and procedures of tracking ticks are more advanced in central Europe and the former Soviet Union. Europe's and Russia's head start in the surveillance of *Ixodes*-transmitted diseases was the consequence of their long experience with tick-borne viral encephalitis. In the United States, the need for better surveillance of Lyme disease unfortunately comes when many state and local governments have less financial ability to undertake this research, because of budget constraints and other demands. The federal government also has fewer resources for this activity; between 1992 and 1994, for example, the Centers for Disease Control unit that tracks and investigates Lyme disease had a 20-percent reduction in staff positions.

In the next chapter we turn away from vectors, hosts, and reservoirs, and return to Julia, Werner, Catherine, and Roy, whose stories we took up in Chapter 1. Their stories lead us to an explanation of how Lyme disease is diagnosed.

How Do You Know That You Have Lyme Disease?

$$\boxed{4}$$

- After Julia and her mother noticed Julia's unusual rash, they went to the clinic and told the pediatrician about Julia's rash and headache. When the pediatrician saw the rash she thought that it probably indicated Lyme disease. She had been in practice in the area for several years, and the shape, size, and color of the rash on Julia's leg were similar to what she had seen in other cases of Lyme disease at that stage. But she wanted more evidence before starting treatment, so she asked more questions, performed a physical examination, and did some blood tests.

  As Julia and her mother answered the pediatrician's questions, the pediatrician learned that Julia often played outside, in a grove of trees near her home, and that the family frequently saw deer around the neighborhood. Sometimes, when Julia and her brothers came in from playing, their parents would find small ticks on the children's clothing or skin.

  When the pediatrician examined Julia, she found some swollen lymph nodes in her groin. She also discovered a second red patch on Julia's back which was so faint as to be hardly noticeable. Julia was alert, and her neck was not stiff or painful, so the pediatrician decided not to do a spinal tap. But she did take a blood sample, which was examined later that afternoon in the clinic's laboratory. There was a normal number of red and white blood cells in the blood, and the screening test for mononucleosis ("mono") was negative. Julia's urine was also examined and showed no sign of kidney or bladder infection. After seeing the test results, which ruled out other diseases and disorders, the pediatrician told Julia and her mother that Julia had Lyme disease.

- By the time Werner reached the hospital at his medical school, the pain in his arm was worse. He was not sure which bothered him more: the pain in his arm or the embarrassment of having one side of his face droop. In the emergency room, a neurologist—a specialist in diseases of the nervous system—was called in to see Werner. After examining Werner, the neurologist first assured him that he was not having a stroke. The specialist also thought that multiple sclerosis was unlikely, but in order to get a better idea of what was going on, he recommended doing a lumbar puncture (a spinal tap) to obtain a sample of the fluid that bathed Werner's brain.

For the lumbar puncture Werner lay on his side on the examination table and curled up. The neurologist disinfected a small region of the exposed skin on his back, inserted a thin, hollow needle through the bones of Werner's back into the spinal canal, removed about a teaspoonful of clear, colorless *cerebrospinal* fluid through the needle, and sent it to the laboratory. The report soon came back from the lab saying that the fluid contained an abnormally large number of white blood cells as well as an abnormally large amount of protein; these findings indicated that Werner's nervous system was inflamed. There were several possible explanations for this inflammation, and Lyme disease was one of them.

By questioning Werner, the physician learned that he often walked through the forests surrounding Vienna. This was an area known to contain the ticks that carry the Lyme disease spirochete. However, Werner was sexually active, so syphilis was a possibility. Tests on Werner's blood and spinal fluid could help the physician tell whether Werner's problem was Lyme disease or syphilis.

Some of the tests were completed that same day, in the same hospital. For some of the other tests, the fluid samples had to be sent to a laboratory in another city. When the results arrived a few days later, they showed that Werner had antibodies in his blood and spinal fluid to the spirochetes that cause Lyme disease, but not to the spirochetes that cause syphilis. The neurologist concluded that Werner probably had Lyme disease.

■ When her physician saw Catherine limping into the office, he began to make a mental list of what could be causing her to have pain in her leg. In Arizona, Lyme disease was not high on the list. Most likely it would be osteoarthritis, the thinning of the joint lining after years of wear and tear. But after hearing that she had never had a problem with her knee or any other joints before, the physician knew he had to go further down the list.

Among other questions, he asked whether she had traveled out of the state that year. She said that she had been in Hawaii at Christmas time, and that the previous summer she had spent two weeks with her sister on Long Island, New York. His ears perked up when he heard about the visit to the coast of the northeastern United States, a place where he knew that Lyme disease could be contracted.

Except for her swollen knee, Catherine had a normal physical exam. The physician obtained fluid from the knee by inserting a small needle into the space around the joint. When the fluid was examined in the laboratory, no evidence was found of a staphylococcus bacterial infection (commonly called a "staph" infection); nor was there any sign of gout. These were other diagnoses the physician had considered. Now Lyme disease moved up on the list of possibilities.

The physician ordered a blood test for Lyme disease and one for rheumatoid arthritis. In a few days the results came back: "positive" for Lyme disease, "negative" for rheumatoid arthritis. To help confirm the diagnosis, the physician asked the laboratory to run a "Western blot" test for Lyme disease on the same blood sample. That test was also positive. There was little doubt about the diagnosis now.

When told that she had Lyme disease, Catherine said that she had heard of it but that she thought you could only get it from hiking or camping. She had spent almost all her vacation around the vacation house, on the beach, or on the golf course. And she hadn't seen any ticks. When the physician asked her about insect bites, though, she remembered having had what she thought was an insect bite on the back of her leg. The large red spot had cleared up by the time she returned to Phoenix.

■ In the cardiac care unit of the hospital, Roy's cardiologist said that he was frankly stumped about what could have caused Roy's heart to beat so irregularly. There was no evidence of a true heart attack, which leaves permanent damage. But the electrocardiogram showed that there was mild temporary damage to the heart.

The cardiologist thought that Roy probably had a virus infection that had settled in the heart. There was not much to be done about that; Roy would probably get over the damage with time. Another possibility was Lyme disease. Since Lyme disease is treatable, it certainly was a diagnosis worth pursuing. To be on the safe side, then, the physician ordered a blood test for that disorder.

Over the next two days Roy's heart condition remained stable, but he had a low-grade fever that suggested a continuing infection. When the Lyme disease blood test came back positive, the cardiologist called in an infectious disease specialist as a consultant. The physician reviewed the case notes first and saw that Roy lived in Westchester County. Later she asked Roy about the neighborhood he lived in and learned that it was suburban, with forests backing up to many of the yards.

It turned out that Roy's son had developed Lyme disease two summers before this. He had developed a rash that looked like a red target, and he was treated right away by their family physician. The infectious disease specialist also learned that Roy's pet dog had become lame in the last two weeks. Roy himself had felt ill with what he thought was a "summer flu" a few weeks ago, but he did not recall any rash, joint pains, or nerve weakness. The consultant concluded that this was Lyme disease.

As the stories of Julia, Werner, Catherine, and Roy demonstrate, making the diagnosis of Lyme disease can be easy or hard. But even in the cases where diagnosis was difficult, a diagnosis was eventually made. And in each of these cases the physician was confident about the diagnosis, either at the first visit or after the laboratory results were received.

Is this how things usually turn out when someone has Lyme disease? Is the diagnosis usually so clear-cut? And are physicians always so confident that the diagnosis is accurate? The short answer is no. But a more complete consideration of the question produces an answer that is more optimistic and that identifies which aspects of Lyme disease medical science *is* reasonably certain about.

In each of the stories related above, the diagnosis was made by the practitioner. A commonly held assumption has been that a sick person goes to the physician for a diagnosis and treatment and is, in many ways, completely in the physician's hands. Although this is still the most common situation, many people now feel able to make a diagnosis themselves, and even if they aren't able to initiate their own treatment, they can at least present their conclusions to a physician or other health care provider, who still has the power of the prescription pad.

Is the latter approach reasonable with regard to Lyme disease? Can a person reliably make the diagnosis of Lyme disease in himself or herself or in a family member or friend? The short answer is yes. But there are many pitfalls to this approach, not the least of which is the possibility that other, perhaps more serious diagnoses could be overlooked. And the laboratory tests that can be so important in confirming a diagnosis are still available only to physicians.

Making a Medical Diagnosis

Before going into detail about how Lyme disease is diagnosed, it may be helpful to review the steps that physicians and other practitioners follow in order to make a diagnosis. This process is often compared to the process of solving a crime, but while the two activities have much in common, there are also several differences.

One similarity is the drawing up of a list of "suspects" for the crime or illness. Just as the police officer may bring in for questioning people who by virtue of their records may be suspected of having committed the crime, so the physician produces what is known as a "differential diagnosis," a list of specific diseases, in order of probability, to be further considered. This list may be short—as short as one item—if the diagnosis is clear, or it may be long, if the cause of the illness is obscure. Catherine's physician began to make such a list when he saw her walking down the hall. The list is refined, resorted, and reevaluated as additional information is accumulated.

To gather information about the patient and the illness, the physician generally takes the following steps: he or she first takes a medical history, next performs a physical examination, and finally orders any x-rays or other laboratory tests that may be appropriate.

Taking a history, as the name implies, involves developing an understanding of the sequence of events that led the person to visit the practitioner's office. The patient tells the physician about the symptoms he or she is experiencing, when they started, whether they have gotten worse, whether they are continuous or intermittent, what makes them worse, and what if anything relieves them. The physician may ask the patient specific questions in order to get information he or she needs. If the physician does not know the patient, he or she will ask the patient about other conditions the patient has now or has had in the past, as well as allergies or sensitivities to medicine, and any diseases that may run in the family.

In an ideal encounter between physician and patient there is enough time for a thorough history to be taken. Unfortunately, this is not always the case, and so, sometimes, the "database" on which the physician must base a diagnosis is incomplete. It is always helpful when the patient brings in written notes about what happened and about the present symptoms. This information is likely to be more accurate than information carried in one's head, and it makes it less likely that anything of importance will be overlooked. Such notes should include the names and dosages of any medicines that are presently being taken. If a person is seeing a new physician, it is helpful if the person brings along medical records documenting previous treatment; this can save time and reduce repetition of questions and laboratory tests.

The next step is the physical examination, which can range in extent from limited to comprehensive, depending on the complexity of the illness and whether the physician has seen the patient previously—and, if so, how long ago. Usually the physician asks additional questions while performing the exam. During the exam, too, the patient may mention other symptoms that seem unrelated to the present problem but may nonetheless turn out to be important.

After completing the physical examination the physician usually has a pretty good idea of what is going on. Or, if the diagnosis is not crystal clear, at least he or she has eliminated many diagnoses from further consideration. Often the physician will decide at this point that no laboratory tests or x-rays are needed, and will dispense either appropriate treatment or reassurance—or both. Sometimes, though, the recommendation will be that the patient have some diagnostic tests: an x-ray of some kind, or another procedure, such as an electrocardiogram.

These tests may be ordered to confirm a diagnosis that seems likely, given the information provided by the history and physical examination. Alternatively, they may be ordered because it is not at all clear what is going on. In this case, the physician depends on the test results to inform the decision-making process. An example of this situation is a culture of the blood for microorganisms in a case of fever lasting for weeks. In such cases the physician may suspect that the patient has an infection but may have little evidence to go on in determining what and where the infection is.

Sometimes tests are done not so much to make a diagnosis as to determine whether the patient is a good candidate for a new medication or an operation. For instance, if it is discovered, through testing, that a person has diseased kidneys, it may be necessary to modify the patient's dose of a medication. Or a chest x-ray before surgery may reveal lung disease that would increase the person's risk if he or she were put under general anesthesia; such a finding may result in the surgery being canceled or the approach to anesthesia being modified.

Current conditions in medical practice make it more likely that physicians will use and depend on laboratory tests and other procedures. These conditions include time pressures, which make it difficult for the physician to spend the appropriate amount of time talking to the patient, and the perceived threat of medical malpractice suits. The legal threat may cause the physician to order tests to rule out even diseases that are relatively unlikely in light of the medical history and physical examination. This behavior is justified on the grounds that if a serious disease is missed the physician may be sued, even if it can be agreed that the disease was very unlikely to begin with. The other condition encouraging the use of tests—the time pressure that discourages spending time with patients—has arisen in part because physicians usually receive higher compensation for performing a test or procedure than for taking time with the history, performing the physical exam, and explaining treatments.

Physicians also depend on laboratory tests because they are trained to do so in medical school and as interns and residents. The ultimate aim of medical diagnosis, as it has usually been taught, is to identify a specific disease in the patient. "Disease" in this context means a defined abnormality in the tissues of one or more organs. Once a disease diagnosis has been made, it is reasoned, a specific treatment can be applied.

If a microscope could be used to examine the patient's tissue (and this is possible in certain circumstances, such as when pieces of tissue are removed for a biopsy), the examination would reveal differences between a diseased person and a "normal" person. One example of such a difference would be the presence of large numbers of white cells in the liver. These are signs of a type of *hepatitis*, the general name for a disease that involves inflammation of the liver.

But because blood and other fluids provide a window to the body (a way to see inside the body), tests of the blood can often establish conclusively that the patient has a disease—or doesn't have a disease—even without direct examination of tissue samples. To continue with the above example, a blood test showing elevation of an enzyme (a type of protein) produced by the liver would be an indication that liver cells are damaged. In effect, they have become leaky.

Physicians who are faced with a patient's bewildering collection of symptoms are in some ways relieved when a "disease" is discovered through a laboratory or x-ray procedure. They can now turn to the impressive armamentarium of medicines or surgeries available to deal with most problems. In achieving the goal of specific disease diagnosis, the physician has successfully followed the lead of his mentors. But there is an inherent danger in following the model too strictly: the "disease" may be managed "by the book" (in this case, the medical textbook), regardless of what the patient is actually experiencing.

More and more people are recognizing that illness and the perception of illness are affected by many factors besides the malfunctioning organ. These include cultural and personal issues surrounding what an illness means to a patient. People express their diseases, their cell abnormalities, in different ways. In one patient a "disease" may be diagnosed and the correct treatment given, but the patient still feels ill. When the same "disease" is diagnosed in another patient, and the same treatment is given, the outcome may be very different.

As we shall see, this often happens when the diagnosis of Lyme disease is made.

As may be obvious by now, a diagnosis—what is written down in the medical chart or hospital record—comes in different degrees of certainty. Some diagnoses, typically those at the beginning of the work-up, are provisional. They may be changed when conflicting information is obtained or after what would seem to be an appropriate course of treatment fails. In other cases—and this may occur either sooner or later—the diagnosis is definite.

A definite diagnosis may be arrived at in several ways. Sometimes the story the patient offers or the physician elicits is so typical of a particular condition that further examinations are only confirmatory. An example of this would be a history of migraine headaches. The physician can make a diagnosis at a high level of certainty just from hearing about the patient's headaches and the pattern of headaches. In other cases the disease may be suspected from the patient's story, but it is the physical exam that supplies the proof. Examples of this are asthma, confirmed when the physician listens to the chest and hears wheezes, and many diseases of the skin, which is an "organ" that is accessible to the eyes and touch of the physician.

Finally, as noted above, a definite diagnosis may in some cases only be made after tissue taken from the patient has been examined. This examination can be achieved through biopsy, in which a tissue sample is obtained with a minor surgical procedure. A woman may have a lump in a breast, discovered by herself or her physician, or by mammogram, but it is only through a breast biopsy that the diagnosis of cancer can be made or ruled out.

When it comes to Lyme disease, a definite diagnosis may be made at any one of the three steps in the diagnostic process: the history, the physical examination, or laboratory tests. Often, however, a diagnosis of Lyme disease is not definite. Instead, the diagnosis falls into the category of "probable" or "possible."

Diagnosing Lyme Disease
The History

Figuring the odds. One of the enduring aphorisms of medicine (in North America, at least) is this: If you hear hoofbeats outside the house, think of horses and not zebras. Indeed, to denigrate a diagnosis made by a student, trainee, or colleague, one needs only to call it a "zebra," meaning that the diagnosis is very unlikely in that person in that locale. For example, a diagnosis of malaria in a person with a fever who has never been outside of Minnesota is a zebra. It is remotely possible that the person has malaria, perhaps contracted from a blood transfusion. However, it would be inappropriate to inflate the odds for a diagnosis of malaria, particularly if doing so meant that a more likely and more treatable diagnosis was overlooked. If all the "remotely possible" diagnoses for every illness were explored or treated, the hospital bill would be huge and the patient overwhelmed with tests and medicines.

Lyme disease, like malaria, does not occur everywhere in the world. Nor, as discussed in Chapter 2, is it found in every part of the United States. Even within states that report many cases of the disease, the risk of contracting it varies greatly by locale. In many places, a person's chances of getting Lyme disease are zero. Essentially the only way that a person can get the disease is by living in or visiting a place where ticks with the spirochetes exist. For example, although Westchester County, New York, reports many cases of the infection each year, a resident of that county who stays in strictly urban areas, where deer are not present, has little or no risk of Lyme disease.

Today, Lyme disease ticks and *B. burgdorferi* spirochetes appear to be spreading to areas where they have never been reported before. But this spread is comparatively slow compared with the spread of the virus that causes influenza, for example. It is also possible that infections that resemble Lyme disease occasionally occur in parts of the country with different kinds of ticks. But this situation seems to be limited at this time to the south-central and southeastern states.

What all of this is leading up to is a recognition of the importance of estimating risk. Estimating the individual's risk of getting Lyme disease is an important part of diagnosing the disease. Estimating risk is much like estimating the odds of winning a lottery. If you have a thousand tickets for the next drawing, the probability that you are holding a winning ticket is higher than if you only had one ticket. If the patient has been living in or has visited an area in which the infection is known to occur, then he or she is holding a fair number of Lyme disease "tickets." Additional "tickets" are obtained by spending time out of doors in areas where deer have been observed. When a diagnosis of Lyme disease is being considered in a person living or working in an area where the infection has not been confirmed, then that person's travel history becomes important.

Without uncovering evidence that the patient has either lived in or visited an area where the disease is present, the physician should discard a diagnosis of Lyme disease. One would think that this is common sense, and so it is surprising to learn that the opposite course frequently is taken—that is, that Lyme disease is often considered a "horse" when "zebra" would be more appropriate. The unfortunate result is that the Lyme disease label is pinned on someone. More unfortunate still is the fact that this prevents the correct diagnosis from being made.

Listening to the symptoms. What would lead a physician to think of Lyme disease to begin with? Before the odds of infection are estimated, the proverbial light bulb in the brain must go on. The stories of our four patients provide examples of how this happens. In each case the physician began thinking of Lyme disease as a diagnosis when he or she listened to and examined the patient. With Julia it was after seeing the suggestive skin rash. Werner had weakness of his face muscles and pain in his arm. Catherine had an unexplained arthritis of the knee. Roy's heart inexplicably slowed down. Certainly there may be other causes of these conditions, but Lyme disease ended up on the differential diagnosis list for each of the four people. It was initially high for Julia and low for Catherine, principally because Julia lived in an area where Lyme disease was known to occur and Catherine did not.

There are some symptoms that are either highly uncommon or don't exist at all for Lyme disease. If these symptoms occur, another diagnosis should be considered instead of Lyme disease, or at least in addition to it. These include but are not limited to the following: shaking chills from a high fever; sweating at night that drenches the bedclothes; unexplained loss of more than a few pounds; diarrhea with several bowel movements a day; recurrent pain in the abdomen; pain during urination; blood in the stool; a persistent cough; heartburn; and nasal discharge.

There are other symptoms that are not necessarily indicative of Lyme disease. People with arthritis from Lyme disease, for example, usually do not have their greatest pain or swelling in their hands or feet. Severe back or neck pain is uncommon. In addition, patients with involvement of the nervous system from Lyme disease usually do not have seizures or fits, marked incoordination of their limbs, inability to speak or understand, or loss of control over bladder or bowels. People with Lyme disease of the heart, at least in its early stage, usually do not have pain in the chest or built-up fluid in the lungs or legs; nor do they cough up blood.

After this litany of what Lyme disease is *not* and the limitations of diagnosis by history, it is helpful to remember that a patient's history can be so suggestive of Lyme disease that the diagnosis could be made just by hearing it. One such history concerns a person who developed a targetlike skin rash in the late spring and a few weeks later had weakness on the side of his face, pain and swelling of his joints, and a profound slowing of the heartbeat. Other than Lyme disease, there are few (if any) diseases that this could be. If everyone who was infected with *Borrelia burgdorferi* showed up with symptoms like this, then the diagnosis of Lyme disease would be quick, easy, and cheap. Unfortunately, such stories are unusual. More commonly, the rash was either not noticed or not remembered. Or if the rash was observed, only one of the typical complications followed its disappearance. In such cases the physical exam and laboratory tests assume more importance.

The Physical Exam: The Skin Rash

Julia's physician thought that it was unlikely that the child's rash was caused by anything other than Lyme disease. The physician's confidence about the diagnosis derived in part from the fact that she had seen so many Lyme disease rashes. Someone with less experience might have been stumped, at least initially. There are many causes of a red rash on one or more parts of the body, and often the cause of a rash cannot be readily discovered. In these cases the rash is treated empirically—that is, with "whatever works." Sometimes it may be treated with cortisone or steroid ointment, at other times with an antifungal cream. Still, in a case of Lyme disease, there are features of the rash that suggest erythema migrans, even to a practitioner who has never seen a case before.

An important consideration for the diagnosis is time of year. A rash appearing in the middle of winter in New York or Massachusetts is unlikely to be erythema migrans. In the great majority of cases of Lyme disease with a rash, the rash appears in the late spring, the summer, or the early fall. There may be exceptions to this in warmer climates, but the frequency of the disease is still highest by far in areas with four seasons. Lyme disease starts with a tick bite, and ticks are active only during certain periods of the year. In general, the more northerly the latitude, the more restricted the tick-bite season.

The rash starts at a place where a tick embedded. Sometimes a small tick engorged with blood may still be present. Many people develop a small, slightly elevated area of redness around a tick bite or an embedded tick. This can occur with many types of ticks and in the absence of any spirochetes. In these cases the body is reacting to the tick itself, or to substances the tick left behind. Typically, this limited rash—usually smaller than a quarter—appears within a day or two of the tick bite and then fades over the course of a few days. As discussed previously, some tick bites become infected with other types of bacteria that are already present on the person's skin. The rash and swelling, the cellulitis, from these "staph" or "strep" bacteria can spread very rapidly and need immediate medical attention. Some of these infections can become life-threatening. Cellulitis may follow other small breaks in the skin besides a tick or insect bite. High fever and a painful rash are more suggestive of cellulitis than of erythema migrans.

The rash of erythema migrans begins like a reaction to the tick bite itself—that is, as a small area of redness. The onset of erythema migrans is later than that of the tick bite reaction, however: it occurs three to fourteen days after the bite instead of one to three days. Erythema migrans is also less likely than bite reactions to itch. In fact, if the rash appears in an area such as the back of the leg, where a person does not usually look, it may be missed entirely. A tip-off feature of the rash of erythema migrans is its ringlike appearance: a red circle enclosing a paler center. As described above, there may be another ring within, giving the rash the appearance of a target. Some Lyme disease rashes are solidly red with only a hint of clearing in the center. But erythema migrans rashes are not always circular: triangular or almond-shaped rashes can occur during the early infection.

What the early Lyme disease rash of erythema migrans usually is *not* is scaly, crusty, or blistery. Hives or welts are not typical and suggest another diagnosis, such as an allergic reaction to an insect bite or sting. A rash on the soles of the feet or the palms of the hands is very unusual in Lyme disease. The combination of a skin rash and blisters or ulcers of the mouth is not Lyme disease. Neither is a skin rash of the head with loss of hair.

A common misconception about the rash of Lyme disease is that it can commonly return during late disease, months to years after the onset of the disease. Many people wonder if they have Lyme disease because they have heard or read that people with the disorder have the symptoms they are experiencing: a rash and joint pains, perhaps with fatigue, headache, and other symptoms as well. During the early phase of Lyme disease, people may have the rash and feel achy all over. They may even experience a return of the rash with multiple red patches or "targets" when joint pains begin, in the first weeks of the infection. This is the result of the spirochetes spreading, through the blood, to other areas of the skin. But the combination of either joint pains and a rash or extreme fatigue and a rash would not be expected to occur months or years later. If people with true Lyme arthritis do get a rash later in the disease, it is more likely for another reason, such as an allergic reaction to a medicine.

The only skin rash from Lyme disease that lasts for months to years is usually known by its tongue-twisting Latin designation, *acrodermatitis chronica atrophicans.* The name essentially means a long-lasting rash of the arms and legs that leaves the skin thin and wrinkled. This rash may evolve directly from erythema migrans, or it may emerge after a disease-free interval. The involved skin may be reddened, but overall the rash resembles an old burn. The appearance of acrodermatitis is not so unique that the diagnosis of Lyme disease could be made just from the presence of this rash. Almost all cases of acrodermatitis have been reported from Europe and Russia. It is rare, if it occurs at all, in North America.

The other skin condition that is very suggestive of infection with a Lyme disease spirochete is *lymphocytoma.* Like acrodermatitis, it is much more common in Europe than in North America. Lymphocytoma is a deep reddening and hardening of one of the ear lobes or of the areola around a nipple. Many people remember a tick bite at those sites. Ticks in those locations would be hard to miss.

The Physical Exam: The Rest of the Body

The remainder of the physical exam may reveal other signs of infection with *B. burgdorferi,* but these signs are not as specific for Lyme disease as the rashes erythema migrans or lymphocytoma. There is nothing unique to Lyme disease about a weakness in facial muscles, swelling and pain of a joint, or a slowing of the heartbeat. For each of these disorders there may be other explanations. Of course, if all three of these conditions occur at the same time or in succession, then Lyme disease is the number one suspect. But, as already mentioned, such a case seldom appears.

The examining physician may discover other abnormalities during the physical exam. In the early stages of the disease, when a rash is usually present, these include a redness at the back of the throat; swelling of some lymph nodes of the neck, armpits, or groin; and redness of the eyes. If there is a fever in Lyme disease, it is usually not higher than 102°F. A temperature higher than this is probably caused by another infection or condition. The pulse may be more rapid than normal, especially if there is a mild fever. If the pulse is much slower than usual, the heart may be involved. Blood pressure seldom is much higher or lower than usual.

When the patient or his or her family expresses concerns about forgetfulness, inability to concentrate, sleep difficulties, or irritability, the patient's "mental status" is checked. At that point in the examination the physician asks the patient to remember objects and to perform some mental and written tasks. Such tests commonly demonstrate that concerns about the patient's supposedly failing abilities are groundless; as a consequence, these tests are often reassuring. In other cases real impairments are revealed which may be an indication of brain involvement in the Lyme disease infection. Because depression can produce the same symptoms and mental deficits that Lyme disease causes, the physician may also assess the patient's self-esteem and ask the patient whether he or she has been feeling inadequate or despondent, whether he or she has noticed any loss of interest in life's pleasures, and whether there have been any thoughts of suicide.

Some findings on the physical exam would be so unusual for Lyme disease on its own that other diagnoses must be considered. These include swelling or marked tenderness of the abdomen; a new murmur of the heart; enlargement of the liver; fluid in the lungs; and swelling and tenderness of the joints of the hands or feet.

Do-It-Yourself Diagnosis?

Lyme disease is seldom if ever discovered during a routine physical examination. If a person has been feeling well and goes to the physician for a check-up, the physician might detect high blood pressure, a breast lump, or an enlarged prostate; but the physician is unlikely to "find" Lyme disease during such an examination.

Usually, the first step toward a diagnosis of Lyme disease is taken by a person who concludes that something is wrong with himself or herself or his or her child. Such a person might then seek out a medical expert to identify exactly what the problem is. But we diagnose for ourselves many common illnesses and disorders, such as a head cold, a sprained back, or a temporary headache, and we decide how to treat the problem, as well. Even when we do seek out a practitioner, we usually have localized the disorder to a specific part of the body. Many times we suspect that we know what the diagnosis will be, especially if we've had the same or a similar illness in the past. Sometimes we seek out a physician because we are afraid that we have something seriously wrong with us, such as cancer.

How do we conclude that the pain in our stomach is cancer, or that the pressure in our chest after climbing the stairs is heart disease? We experience pain, shortness of breath, nausea, cramps, "pins and needles" sensations, and so on. We do not "feel" cancer itself. That is a concept that is learned, perhaps from our parents, perhaps in school or from the news media. In the same way, people with *B. burgdorferi* infection experience one or more of a variety of symptoms, but there is nothing in the sensations themselves that says, "This is Lyme disease." It is only after we have read or heard about Lyme disease that a particular symptom or particular groups of symptoms suggest to us that diagnosis. This tendency to attribute our bodily dysfunctions to a specific disease—this tendency to diagnose ourselves—is a double-edged sword.

The benefit of self-diagnosis is that a disease that is treatable is appropriately paid attention to, perhaps at a point when the symptoms themselves are not particularly disabling. A woman feels a pea-sized mass in her breast and justifiably wonders if this is cancer. This prompts a call to her gynecologist, and a mammogram is performed. A man has transient pain in his chest and left arm and rightly wonders whether he is at risk of a heart attack. A treadmill stress test later that week reveals poor blood flow in his heart's arteries. A Connecticut resident with knee pain and swelling four months after an episode of skin rash wonders whether this could be the same tick disease that his neighbor had last year. So he asks his physician whether this could be Lyme disease, and the physician agrees that it might be and orders a blood test. It is positive, and antibiotics are started that week. A person who suspects that he or she has Lyme disease may even go directly to someone who has a reputation of being highly skilled at taking care of this disorder.

A downside of self-diagnosis, even for health care professionals, is the tendency to force the symptoms to fit one disease rather than dealing with the symptoms as they are and trying to find an appropriate diagnosis among the many possibilities. Once the idea of Lyme disease is raised as an explanation for a person's physical problems, then it is tempting to fit all the symptoms into this diagnostic bag. It may be human nature to seek an explanation for the bad things that happen to us. For many people, any diagnosis, even an inaccurate one, seems to be preferable to uncertainty. Some physicians are equally ill at ease without a specific diagnosis to act upon. In these situations the patient's proposal of the diagnosis of Lyme disease is accepted by the physician, and antibiotic therapy follows. This is fine if the person really did have an infection with *B. burgdorferi*. But what if the person did not?

One outcome of such a diagnostic error is the phenomenon of *non-disease*. This is the identification of disease when it is not actually present. Examples of non-disease are the labeling of a normal variation of mood as a psychiatric disease, or the diagnosis of a heart disorder in a child who has an inconsequential heart murmur. A person or his physician has a check list of the possible symptoms of Lyme disease and concludes that occasional joint aches, fatigue, and headache are Lyme disease instead of the effects of a stressful lifestyle that they are.

One consequence of a non-disease diagnosis is further testing and investigations; these have their costs in terms of money, test complications, and mental anguish. In a case of "non–Lyme disease" there may also be unwanted side effects from antibiotic therapy. An insidious effect of the non-disease phenomenon occurs when someone who is actually in good health assumes the role of a sick person. A child erroneously diagnosed with heart disease may needlessly be restricted from physical play; a family with a member said to have Lyme disease may unnecessarily avoid outdoor activities.

There is an even more unfortunate outcome of a false diagnosis of Lyme disease: when a false diagnosis is settled on, diagnosis of a serious disease, such as cancer or major depression, may be overlooked. In this case, not only has the wrong diagnosis been made—with the repercussions of that error—but the patient will miss the opportunity to receive proper treatment.

One way to minimize incorrect diagnoses of Lyme disease is for the physician to listen to the patient's story and to place the patient's illness into the context of the risk of exposure to disease-bearing ticks. A check-list approach with inordinate emphasis placed on non-specific symptoms such as fatigue should be avoided. The temporal sequence of events is also very important in the history: the arthritis should follow the skin rash and not the other way around. Complementary to a thoughtful and skillfully performed history and physical is the appropriate and prudent application of laboratory tests. A common cause of this misdiagnosis is an error in interpreting the results of blood tests. Blood tests and other diagnostic procedures are considered in the next chapter.

Using Laboratory Tests
to Diagnose Lyme Disease

5

Having a blood test during a visit to a physician is fairly routine these days, and hospitalized people are invariably subjected to a series of visits by the phlebotomist, who draws blood for testing of various kinds. Two centuries ago physicians also took blood from their patients, in a well-meant but generally misguided therapy called bloodletting. Even during much of this century, though, little information could be gained from examining a sample of blood. In the first few decades of the twentieth century physicians seldom knew what to test for or how to interpret the test results.

Contrast that with the situation today. Over the last few decades the variety of blood tests has been increasing almost exponentially. If a substance or cell in the blood has been identified and named, it very likely can be measured in a medical laboratory. The types of blood tests now number in the hundreds.

There's no doubt that these new tests, or *assays*, as they are usually called in medical texts, have improved the quality of our health care. Precise diagnosis can often be made by testing the blood or another body fluid; in addition, the severity of illness can be assessed, the function of individual organs can be measured, and levels of medications in the blood can be monitored. Not only a diagnosis but also optimal therapy can be determined on the basis of the laboratory test results. Even so, tests are not the end-all or be-all for diagnosis. To ensure the best medical care, laboratory tests should complement, not replace, the results from the history and the physical examination. When it takes less time—and is more remunerative—to fill out a laboratory request slip than to take a thorough history, there is a danger of physicians becoming overly dependent on laboratory tests for making diagnoses.

Despite the danger of overusing or becoming overdependent on blood tests, the value of these tests, as noted, is considerable, for they can reveal the presence of a disease not previously known or suspected. When blood is tested for various diseases without there being a good reason to suspect (on the basis of the person's medical history or a physical examination) that the person has any of these diseases, it is said that the blood is being "screened" for disease. As the word *screening* implies, this is like putting a lot of gravel from a stream bed into wire mesh and looking for the rare gold nugget, only in this case the goal of the search is a diagnostic "answer" to the patient's symptoms.

The cholesterol test that is performed in shopping malls as well as in physicians' offices is an example of a screening test. This test is given to everyone, even people without symptoms, and is intended to identify people with high cholesterol levels who may not have any other indication that they are at high risk of a heart attack or stroke. Another example of a screening test is the infamous blood test that couples still must undergo before getting married in many states. The rationale for this prenuptial check for evidence of syphilis is that this is an infection that can be silent for many years and that can be passed on to one's children; if everyone is screened, the testing process discovers those who have the disease and are therefore in need of treatment. The armed services' requirement that recruits be screened for infection with HIV, the cause of AIDS, is another example of mass screening. Discovery of an undiagnosed case of syphilis or HIV infection in these situations is about as infrequent as discovery of a gold nugget in a slurry screen, but screening has been justified in these situations for public health reasons.

Can a blood test be used to screen for Lyme disease? In many cases the test has served this purpose. Consider the person who has some symptoms that suggest Lyme disease. The physician thinks the chances that the person has the disease are low, yet he or she orders the test anyway. The physician's reasoning may have been something like this: "If the test results are positive, then I have the answer and treatment can be started. But if the results are negative, then at least I made sure that Lyme disease was ruled out as a consideration. Lyme disease is something I don't want to miss, because it's treatable."

This sounds reasonable. But is it? The unexpected finding of Lyme disease in someone with atypical symptoms can be gratifying for both patient and physician. But can we really have our cake and eat it too? Are the tests so accurate that we can accept the laboratory results as proof of Lyme disease even when the findings from the history and the physical examination argue against this diagnosis? What are the benefits and drawbacks to a screening approach to Lyme disease diagnosis?

Answering these and other questions will take us on a tour of the various tests for Lyme disease. We'll see how they are done and how reliable they are. We turn first to the most commonly performed blood test for evidence of Lyme disease, the detection of antibodies in the blood. This will serve as a model for understanding the other laboratory tests described here, including some new and promising tests.

Looking for Antibodies in the Blood

After listening to your story and examining you, the physician may determine that it would be a good idea for you to get a Lyme disease test. This usually means that a sample of your blood will be taken, and then sent to a laboratory for examination. There is no x-ray or ultrasound procedure that by itself will reveal Lyme disease; an electrocardiogram can be used to confirm a diagnosis of a heart attack but not Lyme disease.

Technicians in the laboratory may examine your blood or other body fluid for evidence of the spirochete itself (these tests, called direct tests, are considered later in this chapter). More commonly, however, the laboratory looks for indirect evidence of the infection—namely, the presence in the blood of antibodies to *Borrelia burgdorferi*. Antibodies are the protein molecules that mammals and other vertebrates produce as a defense against infection (see Chapter 1), and in a sense they are tailor-made for the invading microorganism. That is, the antibodies formed in response to an infection are usually unique for that infection.

The antibody test is not foolproof. For one thing, when the laboratory technician finds antibodies to *B. burgdorferi* in the blood (or antibodies to the influenza virus, or to any other infection), this does not necessarily mean that Lyme disease (or influenza) is still active. Antibodies may be present months to years after the infection is over. Another flaw in an antibody test is that the antibodies the laboratory finds may not actually be from a Lyme disease infection. They may be the by-product of another type of infection or type of disease.

When a Lyme disease test is positive but the person does not really have *B. burgdorferi* infection, the reaction is called a *false positive*. A false-positive test may occur when the blood contains antibodies to a spirochete that resembles but is not identical to *B. burgdorferi*. For example, the antibodies may have been formed in response to the spirochete that causes syphilis rather than to the *B. burgdorferi* spirochete. A false-positive test may also result when people have antibodies that are particularly "sticky." (What is behind these and other misleading reactions will be described in more detail along with the specific tests.)

Even with its deficiencies, the antibody test is the laboratory assay most commonly carried out for confirmation of the diagnosis of Lyme disease. Performed by a skilled technician, the test can provide useful information; and interpreted with realistic expectations, the test can make a difference in a diagnostic decision. If you were going to have only one test for Lyme disease, the antibody test would be the best choice. To better appreciate its strengths and weaknesses, let us follow what happens to a blood sample in the process of testing for antibodies to *B. burgdorferi*.

The ELISA Test

For the ELISA test, a tablespoon or two of blood is drawn by a nurse or technician in the physician's office or in a nearby laboratory. Through the thin metal needle in the arm vein, the blood goes into a glass tube with a red rubber stopper. (Some samples of blood may go into tubes with green or blue stoppers, but these are for other types of tests, such as a count of white blood cells.) In the "red top tube," as it is called, the blood clots within a few minutes. The blood cells congeal into a dark red mass, and the straw-colored serum can now be seen. The laboratory technician separates the clotted red blood cells from the serum by spinning the tube rapidly in a centrifuge. The clot goes to the bottom of the tube, and the liquid serum remains on top. The serum is removed, and the red blood cell clot is discarded.

In addition to testing the blood for antibodies to Lyme disease, the laboratory may perform other tests on the serum, such as those that measure the function of the liver and kidneys. It is important to find out whether the kidneys and liver are working well, because the doses of medicines may need to be adjusted if these organs are damaged.

The Lyme disease test may be done in the local hospital or laboratory, but often the local laboratory, after using some of the serum for kidney and liver function tests, will send some serum on to another laboratory, perhaps in the same city or state, or perhaps out of state. If Lyme disease is common in the area, it is likely that the local hospital or lab will do the test. Otherwise, the serum is forwarded to a second laboratory, often called a "reference lab." The reference lab may be a public institution, such as a state health department, or a medical school, or a federal laboratory, though private commercial laboratories are increasingly receiving specimens from across the country and serving as reference laboratories.

Any laboratory doing a Lyme disease assay has the choice of making up its own test "from scratch," or purchasing a commercial kit, which contains in a convenient package all the material for performing the assay. Smaller laboratories are more likely to purchase a kit from a supplier. Some laboratories buy the individual parts of the test and put together the final version themselves. A reference lab is more likely to use its own version of the test.

Regardless of which version is used, the procedure for doing the Lyme disease test is fairly standard. First the serum is diluted twofold, fourfold, eightfold, out to more than a thousandfold. The diluted serum is then put in what looks like a miniature, plastic version of a muffin tin. Stuck to the bottom of each depression, or "well," is a small amount of the Lyme disease spirochete. The bacteria are dead, and in some tests the cells have been broken up into small pieces.

If you have in your serum antibodies to one or more parts of the spirochetes, these will bind to the bottom of the well and will not be

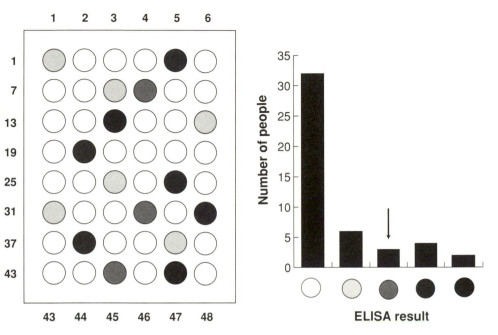

Left: An example of the results of ELISA tests for antibodies to *Borrelia burgdorferi.* There are forty-eight wells for samples in a plastic tray. Each well contains a diluted sample of a different patient's blood. After the test is completed, the wells will have different degrees of a color change. Usually this is yellow or blue; here they are shown as shades of gray. In the example, most of the wells show no color change; they are white. Some wells, such as 47 and 15, show intense color change; here they are black. Patients whose blood shows these strong reactions almost always have or have had infection with *B. burgdorferi.* If they have compatible symptoms and a history of exposure to deer ticks, then the diagnosis of Lyme disease is confirmed. Other patients' blood samples give reactions in the ELISA test that are intermediate in intensity. Some of these persons have been infected with *B. burgdorferi:* others have not. *Right:* A graph showing counts of wells with each shade of color. The cut-off point (indicated by the *arrow*) is the shade or intensity of color above which the test result is considered positive. Just below the cut-off point there may be a few patients who really have *B. burgdorferi* infection; just above it there may be a few people who actually have not been infected. *Drawings by Alan Barbour*

washed away when the wells are washed with a salt-water solution. These bound antibodies can be detected by adding to the wells a second solution, which contains antibodies to antibodies. In other words, the presence of human antibodies stuck to the spirochete parts is revealed by using a special antibody that reacts with, or recognizes, human antibodies. This antibody is generally produced in a goat, sheep, or rabbit by vaccinating these animals with human antibodies. Just as people and animals are immunized with a vaccine to provide them with a ready supply of antibodies against this or that infectious agent, these animals are vaccinated with human antibodies, and therefore they produce antibodies that react to human antibodies.

If the second antibodies, that is, the antibodies to human antibodies, were used just as they came from the animals, it would be difficult to tell if they were present on the bottom of the pan or not. Antibodies are colorless, and the amount that may bind is so small that even if they were blue or red, they would be difficult to detect. The trick used to solve this problem is to link another protein, an enzyme, to the second antibody. This enzyme, like other enzymes, works by changing one chemical compound to another. In this case, the chemical molecule changed is a dye. And when the dye is altered by the enzyme, its color changes. In the most frequently used reactions the chemical compound is changed from white to yellow or blue. Each enzyme molecule can act many times over to change the compounds, making it possible to detect even small amounts of antibodies in the serum.

So the final steps in this antibody test are these: The solution containing the second antibody with its attached enzyme is added to the wells. After an hour or so of incubation, the second antibodies not bound to the bottom of the well are washed away. The presence of the bound second antibodies is then revealed by adding the chemical that turns yellow or blue. The change of color is visible to the eye, but the degree of color change is routinely measured on a machine—the more intense and deeper the yellow or blue, the higher the reading on the machine. ELISA in the name of this test stands for "*enzyme-linked immunosorbent assay.*"

Other Antibody Tests

When the cause of Lyme disease was first discovered more than ten years ago, the first antibody tests performed were not ELISA tests but a test that is performed much the same way that ELISA tests are. In this test, though, the results are determined under a microscope instead of with a plastic tray on a machine. The test is called "indirect immunofluorescence assay," or IFA. Some laboratories still perform this test, although the great majority do ELISA tests. In an IFA test, dead spirochete cells are put on a glass slide; the attached cells are exposed to antibodies in the patient's serum; the unbound antibodies are washed away; and then the bound antibody is revealed through the use of a second antibody. In the case of the IFA, the second antibody has a fluorescent dye attached to it instead of an enzyme. Under ultraviolet light the dye is a brilliant apple green. The technician or physician can tell whether there are antibodies to *B. burgdorferi* in the serum by observing whether the spirochetes on the slide light up under the microscope.

The IFA has the advantage of allowing the technician to see the binding of antibodies to actual cells under the microscope. In the fluorescent patterns there may be subtle but nonetheless telltale signs that indicate that the antibodies bound represent true antibodies to *B. burgdorferi*. The disadvantage of the IFA is that it requires a fair degree of skill and experience to look at the slides and interpret the results accurately. It is easier to train a technician to do ELISA than IFA, and that explains why ELISA tests are done more often than IFA tests.

Several other antibody tests have been described in the medical literature, and some of these are done routinely in some laboratories in the world, but compared with the number of ELISA tests done, the number of these alternative tests done is minuscule. Like the IFA test, most of these tests are technically more complicated and more costly than an ELISA test. Many of these alternative tests offer information that is not provided by the ELISA, however, and it is unfortunate that they are not more widely available.

There is a role for some of these other tests in the laboratory diagnosis of Lyme disease. An advantage of one group of these tests is that the antibodies that are being measured actually attack the spirochetes, revealing how effective the patient's immune response to the invaders is. Either on their own or with help from one or more of the body's other defense mechanisms, the antibodies may either kill the spirochetes or gather them into large, paralyzed clumps. Although these types of tests are generally less sensitive than ELISA for picking up evidence of present or past infection, false-positive results are infrequent.

Pitfalls in ELISA Testing

The results of an ELISA test for antibodies to *B. burgdorferi* may be reported by the laboratory in one of two ways. The first type of test report shows the highest dilution of serum that produces a color change in a well. If the serum was diluted in a ratio of 1:8 (one part of serum to eight parts of saline solution) to begin with and then twofold thereafter, a result of "1:256" means that this dilution of serum produced a defined color change but that a dilution of 1:512 did not. Often such results are reported simply as single figures: "256" or "512," for example. The second, and now more common, type of test report is a numerical value derived by comparing the results obtained with the specific patient's serum to results obtained with sera from people without Lyme disease. For example, let's say that the intensity of the color change in the serum of someone with Lyme disease at a dilution of 1:100 was measured on the machine as 0.74 out of a possible 1.0. On the same day, the serum of someone without Lyme disease produced a value of 0.20. Accordingly, the ratio, or "index" as it sometimes called, is reported as 3.7 (0.74/0.20).

In both types of reporting, the result that is given is one of several possible numbers. The dilution (or titer) of antibody may be 8, 64, 2048, or a value in between. The index, or ratio, may be any value between, say, 0.6 and 5.2. At this stage an interpretation of the raw test result has not been made. The physician could do this himself or herself, but to do so he or she would have to be familiar with Lyme disease testing as well as the disorder. What usually happens is that the laboratory reports whether a certain titer or index value is positive or negative. The laboratory thereby reduces what is actually a point on a scale to a yes or no answer, although sometimes a result in a gray zone between positive and negative is called "borderline" or "indeterminate" by the laboratory.

If a value on a continuous scale is finally reported out as negative or positive, it means that someone, or more likely a committee, has specified a "cutoff point," a test value at or above which the test result is considered to be positive and below which the test result is considered to be negative. How is the cutoff point set? Selecting a cutoff point would be simple if people without Lyme disease showed no reactivity in the assay even with the least diluted samples of serum. But this is not what has been found. On the contrary, a substantial number of healthy people, or "negative controls," as they are known, have had detectable antibodies that bound to spirochete parts in the well of the test plate. These people seldom had titers or color values that were as high as those of Lyme disease patients, but the two groups did overlap. There was no value below which all control sera fell and above which all Lyme disease sera fell.

How could this be? The possibility of a false-positive reaction was discussed above, but that had to do with patients with other diseases. Members of a control group are supposedly free of other diseases. There are three possibilities. The first is that the so-called healthy controls really did have another disease. This could be syphilis, or it could be as innocuous as some mild gum problems. Spirochetes that are not too distantly related to the Lyme disease agent occupy the crevices between teeth and gums. If their numbers get very high, people may develop antibodies to these mouth spirochetes. Some of these antibodies may react with parts of B. burgdorferi, and as a consequence, wells with these sera show color changes, enough perhaps for a false-positive reaction.

The second possible cause of a false-positive reaction among controls is the presence, in the blood, of antibodies that—as mentioned above—are unusually sticky. There are millions of types of antibodies, and some of these have the property of adhering to a variety of surfaces, including the spirochete parts and even the plastic at the bottom of the test well. These sticky antibodies may occur in otherwise normal people, but they are more common in individuals with such autoimmune diseases as lupus erythematosus (often called lupus, or SLE) and rheumatoid arthritis. As the name suggests (the prefix auto- means "self"), in these disorders people have an immune response against their own tissues. Rheumatoid arthritis can be confused in some of its features with the chronic arthritis of Lyme disease, and so a false-positive ELISA reaction based on the presence of sticky antibodies can mean that someone who has rheumatoid arthritis but not Lyme disease may receive inappropriate medical treatment. These types of false-positive reactions may persist indefinitely for some patients; simply repeating the test is of little help.

The third possibility is that some members of the control group actually were infected at some time with *B. burgdorferi*. Infections without the telltale skin rash do occur. When there is no rash, and when the early infection is not followed by arthritis, a nerve disorder, or involvement of the heart, there is nothing to suggest Lyme disease. Infected people may think that they have the "flu" or a "summer virus." The disease, if any was noted at all, passes, while antibodies to the Lyme disease spirochete appear in the blood in response to the mild infection. These antibodies may persist in the blood for months or years. The chance that one of the apparently uninfected controls has had a prior *B. burgdorferi* infection is obviously greater in areas where Lyme disease regularly occurs. That is why negative control sera are best obtained from places far from a Lyme disease area. The only way that residents of such a place can develop *B. burgdorferi* antibodies is by traveling to an area in which Lyme disease transmission occurs.

But what difference does it make if some of the healthy controls had *B. burgdorferi* infections before? Isn't the test designed to determine whether or not someone now has Lyme disease? That is the impression most people have, but the answer, really, is no. Strictly speaking, the test measures antibodies to *B. burgdorferi* cells. Period. Whether these antibodies indicate the presence of an active disease—as opposed to an inactive, past disease—is another matter. Additional information is needed to decide between these two possibilities. That additional data might include a history stating that the only time the patient traveled outside New Mexico (an area without proven Lyme disease transmission) in the last twenty years was three months ago in June, when he spent a month on the New Jersey shore (an area with a lot of Lyme disease). That information suggests that the positive blood test is the result of a recent infection. An important piece of information for interpreting test results might be a report of facial weakness and a targetlike skin rash a few weeks before the blood was drawn from a Minnesota resident. As we have seen, it is usually the case that the history is taken *before* the Lyme disease test is ordered, so these examples are putting the cart before the horse. Such an approach is taken when an apparently healthy person has a positive Lyme disease test, however.

What if someone with a positive Lyme disease test is unable to recount any Lyme disease symptoms or has never been in a place where Lyme disease transmission occurs? In that case, how can we tell whether the test result indicates active or inactive disease? One way is to repeat the test in a few weeks. If the infection is recent, the titer or index of antibodies to *B. burgdorferi* will either rise or fall in the interval between the two tests. Early in the infection the antibodies are rising: the body is responding to the microorganism's presence. After that response has an effect, and the spirochetes are dying or otherwise being held in check, the antibody levels begin to fall. They may continue to fall to undetectable levels, or they may reach a certain lower level and stay there for months, even years. If the infection has been active in the past and is now inactive, or if it is now in the chronic stage, the antibody levels should stay fairly constant from one test to the next. A meaningful change in antibody levels between two or more sequential tests from the same patient is a difference of at least a factor of four. For instance, if the antibody titer in the first test is 128, and it is 512 or higher in a second test four weeks later, this is evidence that the infection is recent. For this approach to be most accurate, the first and second sera should be examined at the same time in the laboratory. Too often, though, the tests are performed on separate occasions. Day-to-day differences in the test itself confound interpretation of these paired results.

A second way to tell in the laboratory if the infection has occurred within a few weeks is to test the blood for a special type of antibody called an immunoglobulin M, or IgM, antibody. IgM antibody is the first type of antibody to appear on the scene of a new infection. The infection may be limited to an area of skin, or it may have spread in the blood to other tissues. As another antibody, the immunoglobulin G, or IgG, rises in the blood, the IgM antibodies peak and then usually fall. While IgM antibodies appear early but recede over the next several weeks, IgG antibodies join the battle later but generally remain on the scene for months or years. Thus, the presence of IgM antibody to *B. burgdorferi* is usually good evidence that an infection is going on *now*. One drawback of the IgM ELISA test, though, is a higher frequency of false-positive reactions than is found with the standard ELISA test. IgM antibodies tend to be more sticky than IgG antibodies. If the IgM antibody test but not the IgG test comes back positive, and other evidence for Lyme disease is not conclusive, it is important to repeat the blood test in a few weeks. In the normal course of infection, the IgM antibody level often will have fallen in the interim, and now the level of IgG antibodies will be higher.

Putting the ELISA Results in Perspective

We return now to the description of how the cutoff point for positive and negative tests is determined. Simply put, the strategy is to maximize the number of true *B. burgdorferi* infections the test picks up and to minimize the number of false-positive reactions. A test's effectiveness in detecting true infections is called its *sensitivity*, and its ability to distinguish present or past true infections from absence of infection is called its *specificity*. On the one hand, if the cutoff point is set too low—for example at an ELISA titer of 32—everybody with *B. burgdorferi* might be identified but many noninfected people might also have "positive" sera. The specificity of the test would be low. (The possible explanations for this are discussed earlier in this chapter.) On the other hand, if the cutoff point is set too high—for example, at 1024—many infections will be missed. In such a situation someone with true Lyme disease whose antibody titer is 256 or 512 will receive a report of a negative ELISA test; the sensitivity is low. The compromise is a cutoff point of, for example, 256, which might detect all but five out of one hundred *B. burgdorferi* infections while erroneously calling positive three sera out of one hundred from people who have never had the infection. In this case the sensitivity is 95 percent. A specificity of 97 percent is obtained by subtracting the false-positive rate, here 3 percent, from 100 percent.

The sensitivity of the most commonly performed type of ELISA is 94 to 98 percent for patients who have had untreated *B. burgdorferi* infections for more than a month or so. The usual specificity under these conditions also is in the range of about 94 to 98 percent. That sounds pretty good, so what is the problem in freely using the test? There is no physical risk to the patient besides a needle stick, and compared with many diagnostic procedures the ELISA test is a bargain. The answer is that the odds that the test will correctly identify an infection are good, even excellent—but only under one circumstance: when the chance of having the disease is high to begin with. When the history and physical examination suggest that the chance of Lyme disease in a given person is low, then the test's accuracy—what is called its *predictive value*—is much lower. That sounds obvious and even undeserving of mention, but the point is important.

Earlier in this chapter we considered the phenomenon of screening for disease and then discussed what it meant if a Lyme disease test result was unexpectedly positive. Maybe we should have asked at that time why the Lyme disease test had been requested in the first place. Perhaps it was routinely requested if there was any chance of Lyme disease. No one, neither patient nor physician, wishes to miss the diagnosis of a disease that is ostensibly treatable with antibiotics. Not only is the opportunity for a cure missed, but riskier therapies might be used instead. Ominously in the background may be the threat of litigation for that error of omission, the overlooked diagnosis. The trick is in deciding what to take seriously. Should it be a one-in-ten chance? One in one hundred? One in one thousand? It may sound coldhearted to be making such determinations when dealing with a person who is ill, but there are important implications here for the individual as well as for "public health" and "society."

The monetary cost of tests is one issue. Each ELISA test costs the patient about $25. If four hundred thousand Lyme disease tests are performed in a year, the total price is $10 million. Until recently, cost has not been much of a disincentive to ordering lab tests: the money usually has not come directly out of the patient's pocket or the physician's office budget. An insurance company, a government, or another third-party payer would pick up all or most of the cost.

Recently, the regulations of the government and the economic forces of managed health care have increased pressure on physicians and patients to control medical care costs, but the primary concern about the inappropriate use of the blood test is still not the monetary cost of the test.

Rather, the greatest concern is the "cost" of overdiagnosing Lyme disease. This cost is measured not just in dollars and cents, but also in the effect overdiagnosis has on peoples' lives. It's one thing for a person to take a drug that is ineffective. What's worse is that the drug may cause side effects; and when intravenous antibiotics are given, the side effects may be severe, as Chapter 6 describes. It is also possible that the person has a different, treatable condition that may be overlooked while the nonexistent "Lyme disease" is being treated.

If we look at two different situations in which a Lyme disease test is ordered, the effect of what can be called the prior odds of having the disease can be appreciated. In the first situation, the patient lives in an area known to have Lyme disease and has had in the past what sounds like a typical skin rash; in addition, the presenting symptoms are compatible with Lyme disease. Before ordering an ELISA test, the physician estimates that the odds that the patient really has Lyme disease are three out of four. Another way of putting it is that the "pre-test probability" of Lyme disease is 75 percent. If there are a hundred such patients with this pre-test probability, then seventy-five would actually have the disease. For this situation and the next we will assume that the ELISA test the physician orders has a sensitivity of 95 percent and a specificity of 95 percent. If one hundred people with these prior odds had this ELISA test, there would be 71 true-positive tests and only one false-positive test. The true-positive results far outnumber the false-positive ones. In this situation, the laboratory test has confirmed the physician's diagnosis. Taking an antibiotic is a very reasonable choice for this patient. There is little chance that this treatment would be carried out in vain.

In the second situation the pre-test probability of Lyme disease is lower. Perhaps the patient has symptoms suggestive of Lyme disease but lives in an area with few or no documented cases of B. burgdor-feri infection. Or the patient resides in a region with a lot of Lyme disease but has only nonspecific symptoms such as fatigue and some joint aches. The physician thinks that the prior odds that the patient actually has Lyme disease are one out of twenty, a pre-test probability of 5 percent. Under this circumstance the report of a positive ELISA test from the lab is less helpful, because it is equally likely that the result is a false-positive as a true-positive reaction. The "post-test" probability is only even odds. Half the time, the patient would not be expected to benefit from Lyme disease treatment. If we assume that the prior odds, or pre-test probability, of true *B. burgdorferi* infection are even lower, say one out of one hundred, then most of the time a positive blood test would be inaccurate.

Improving the Accuracy of the Blood Test

The predictive value of the blood test—for high, low, and in-between pre-test probabilities—could be improved if the test's specificity was higher, that is, if the number of false-positive reactions was reduced. If the specificity went from 94 percent to 99 percent, then a positive test result in the second situation would mean a five-to-one chance, instead of even odds, that the patient really has *B. burgdorferi* infection.

The specificity of the ELISA might be heightened by further tinkering with the test. It is likely that the next generation of ELISA tests, now under development, will have better performance in this respect. To improve the predictive value of the blood test now, another test is used in combination with the ELISA test. This second test is the "Western blot" assay, also known as the "immunoblot" assay. The second name, though less often used than the first, provides a better idea of what the test does. The *immuno-* part of the name suggests immune response and antibodies, and the *-blot* part of the name is just what it suggests: material, in this case proteins, is "blotted" from one sheet to another.

The immunoblot assay is done in several steps. The first involves separating the various proteins of disrupted *B. burgdorferi* cells according to size. This is done in a thin, gelatinlike sheet under the influence of a direct electrical current. Essentially, the smaller proteins move more quickly through the nooks and crannies of the gel than do larger proteins. Once this separation has been achieved, the proteins are blotted in an exact replica to another sheet laid on top of the first. This second sheet can be a refined form of paper or a tougher material such as nylon. From this point on, the procedure is like the ELISA test. That is, the binding of antibodies in the patient's serum to proteins is detected by a second antibody with an enzyme attached. The presence of bound antibodies is revealed by a brown or blue band on the blotted sheet.

The Western blot differs from ELISA assays in that the individual proteins are distributed one-dimensionally over a strip of the sheet instead of occupying a single point at the bottom of an ELISA well. This is significant because the laboratory can tell which of the numerous *B. burgdorferi* proteins the patient has antibodies against. In the ELISA test this is not possible. The Western blot result is reported as the number and identity of the colored bands on the blotted sheet. The Western blot can test for either IgG or IgM antibodies.

A Western blot assay involves more work than an ELISA test, and consequently, it costs more to do. What is the advantage of knowing exactly what proteins someone has antibodies to? The answer brings us back to the problem of antibodies that bind to something in *B. burgdorferi* but actually arose for reasons other than Lyme disease, such as an infection with another type of spirochete. In the ELISA test these "cross-reactive" antibodies cannot be distinguished from antibodies that are the products of an infection with *B. burgdorferi* itself. In the Western blot assay they may not really be distinguished, either. Still, knowing which *B. burgdorferi* protein is being bound by the person's antibodies can be helpful in determining whether the person has Lyme disease.

There are certain proteins of *B. burgdorferi* that are unusual in the world of bacteria and viruses—there seems to be nothing like them among other causes of infectious diseases of people and animals. If an antibody binds to one of these known proteins in the Western blot assay, it is very unlikely that this occurred because of an infection other than Lyme disease. But there are other proteins of *B. burgdorferi* that are similar to proteins of other bacteria, some of which are only distantly related in evolution. Antibodies to these

A B C   A B C

1

2

3

4

For the Western blot test, cells of *Borrelia burgdorferi* are first broken up with a detergent. Most of the proteins of the cell become free and separated from one another in the detergent solution. If this protein solution is then subjected to an electric field, the proteins move through a thin gel according to their sizes. In the detergent the proteins all have the same electric charge. The gel under a micro-scope looks like a sponge with holes and spaces of various sizes. The smallest proteins can get through the spaces quicker than the larger proteins and thus reach the bottom of the gel sooner than the larger proteins. The figure shows three identical lanes, *A, B,* and *C,* in which the proteins of the cells have separated top to bottom in the gel *(front).* The separated proteins are then transferred, or blotted, perpendicularly out of the gel and onto a nylon membrane *(back).* Again, an electric current is used to do this. Once on the membrane, the proteins stick, just like ink on a blotter. The different identical lines of proteins can be separated as strips, which can then be reacted with serum from a patient's blood. For convenience, the *A, B,* and *C* strips have been shown as if they were put back together; but they represent three different patients.

Antibodies that bind to one of the *B. burgdorferi* proteins can be revealed by one of several methods. A type of dye is usually used. The reaction of antibody with a particular protein is called a "band." As can be seen, patients A, B, and C give different Western blot patterns. Patient A has three bands in the blot. Patient B has nine bands, and patient C has eight bands. The bands numbered *1, 2, 3,* and *4* are those in this example that are used to judge whether the test is positive or negative. (Not all or even most of the proteins in *Borrelia burgdorferi* are useful in this way.) For this example we can specify that a positive reaction is any two or more of those four bands. By these criteria, patients B and C have positive Western blots and patient A has a negative test. Patient A does have one band that is among the four, but that is not enough. In general, the more bands a patient's blood shows, the more likely it is to have the right number and kind of bands, but there are exceptions to this. This is one reason there has been confusion and disagreement about the interpretation of the Western blot test. *Drawing by Alan Barbour* proteins of B. *burgdorferi* are more suspect, especially in the absence of antibodies to the more unique proteins. In fact, if the only colored bands in the blot are these proteins that are common to many bacteria, then the Western blot is negative.

The ELISA test might have been positive because of these cross-reactive antibodies. A Western blot–type test picks this up by identifying the proteins that are being bound by antibodies. Conversely, the Western blot also can confirm a positive ELISA result by revealing antibodies bound to the unique and specific B. *burgdorferi* proteins. The Western blot for Lyme disease is considered positive when a combination of certain proteins (bands) is present. By the most commonly used criterion, five proteins out of a list of about ten must be present for a positive IgG test. There is no titer or index; Western blot results are either positive or negative.

The laboratory diagnosis of HIV infection also uses a combination of first an ELISA test and then a Western blot assay if the ELISA is positive. The more expensive Western blot test is reserved for sera already shown to be positive by ELISA. Positive ELISA results often turn out to be false upon follow-up Western blot testing. In most instances the Western blot assay can be run on the same sample of blood, and within a day or two of the ELISA test. At this time the Western blot assay is used as a confirming test only; it does not have a role in *screening* for either HIV infection or B. *burgdorferi* infection. A Western blot test would not be expected to be positive if an ELISA with a suitable cutoff point was negative. If the Western blot test for Lyme disease were to be run routinely, irrespective of the ELISA test result, the patient or insurance company would probably be wasting money.

The Controversy over Seronegative Lyme Disease

The reader may be convinced by now that false-negative antibody tests in chronic Lyme disease are uncommon or rare. This view fits the following paradigm for infectious diseases: when microorganisms are invasive enough to cause sickness of a human being or other animal, detectable antibodies are almost always produced in response to that infection. The exception would be the case of someone who has a defective immune response. Is this paradigm appropriate for Lyme disease? Most if not all Lyme disease experts at academic and governmental institutions would agree that it is. They would point out the infrequent occurrence of false-negative tests in true chronic Lyme disease and would add that even persons without any apparent disease can have measurable amounts of antibodies to *B. burgdorferi* as a result of a past infection.

But there is not universal agreement on this point. Some physicians and other health care providers, as well as some lay people, believe that "seronegative Lyme disease"—meaning late *B. burgdorferi* infection with negative antibody tests—is more common than the preceding discussion, and most Lyme disease researchers, would suggest. This disagreement is not trivial. If we were to accept that seronegative Lyme disease is two or four or ten or fifty times as common as is traditionally accepted, then we would have to accept that the only basis for diagnosis is the history and physical exam.

What problems does this alternative paradigm pose? Consider that, while early Lyme disease with skin rash usually presents few diagnostic dilemmas, chronic or late disease can be confused with many other conditions. An astute diagnostician, following strict clinical and epidemiologic criteria for Lyme disease, would probably have a good batting average, even without confirmatory laboratory testing, in distinguishing "non–Lyme disease" from true chronic Lyme disease. The specificity of his or her clinical diagnosis would be high under these conditions. However, when the physician is asked to identify the presence or absence of Lyme disease among persons who might have less typical cases or less certain exposures, the specificity of clinical diagnosis is lower. The antibody test then becomes a more important variable in eliminating Lyme disease from future diagnostic considerations. Faced with someone who may possibly have Lyme disease—say, someone with a pre-test probability of 10 percent—the physician's usual strategy is to do an antibody test and accept a negative antibody test result as evidence against that diagnosis. We have already considered the dilemma the physician and the patient face if the test is positive under these conditions.

Underpinning this strategy has been the assumption that there is a low false-negative rate for the standard blood tests for chronic disease. According to those with an alternative view, the antibody tests in routine use have lower sensitivity and higher specificity than is generally accepted. By this view, a positive test means that the person has Lyme disease, but a negative test does not rule it out. Under these circumstances the point of testing is altered from ruling out Lyme disease to detecting unsuspected cases. Laboratory tests with low sensitivity but good specificity are more suitable for screening populations than for confirming a diagnosis in an individual patient. The pitfalls of taking a screening approach to *B. burgdorferi* infection were considered earlier in this chapter.

(There is a third view, which remains to be proved. Some cases of so-called seronegative Lyme disease may actually be the result of infections with another microorganism, one that is dissimilar enough to *B. burgdorferi* to give a negative test for antibodies to the Lyme disease agent. This may explain the existence of reports of a disease that looks like Lyme disease from areas in which *B. burgdorferi* transmission to humans does not occur or is rare.)

Laboratory Dependability and Quality Control

In the preceding discussion, there has been an assumption that the blood tests for antibodies were state-of-the-art and were performed competently, and that the sensitivity and specificity were the best that could be expected. The reality is that the sensitivity and specificity of the ELISA and Western blot assays vary greatly between laboratories. In studies in which the same sample of serum was sent to several laboratories and the ELISA results were compared, there was a discouraging lack of consistency between laboratories. Even within the same laboratory different results were obtained when the same serum sample was tested twice. Some laboratories had many more false-positive results than others. Some laboratories had more false-negative results than others.

While we assume that two humans will differ to some degree in the way they interpret an event or in their artistic and athletic performances, we expect scientific laboratories and their machines to be more predictable. How could there be these discrepancies in a laboratory test? One of the problems is that the various laboratories in these surveys were not using the same materials and procedures. Until 1995 there were no national—let alone international—standards for how the tests were to be done.

The basic method for doing the tests was described above; but we've also taken note of the fact that there are differences in such variables as what type of *B. burgdorferi* and what second antibody are used in the test. Also, laboratories generally determine their own cutoff points using groups of control sera that differ from one place to another. If the control sera include samples from some people with inapparent *B. burgdorferi* infections, the cutoff point may be set too high, and if the "positive" control group included some people who really did not have Lyme disease, then the cutoff point may be set too low. If a laboratory buys test kits from a manufacturer, it is dependent on the manufacturer for quality control and for the validity of positive and negative control sera included with the kit.

The Western blot assay is especially prone to differences in performance and interpretation between laboratories. It is more complex than an ELISA test; several different outcomes are possible; the results are less quantitative; a single number is not obtained; faint bands may be difficult to interpret. Rigorous standards need to be applied to make sure that a Western blot performed in one laboratory will give the same result as a blot performed in another testing facility with the same serum sample.

Other Tests: Actual and Possible
The Lymphocyte Proliferation Test

So far we have focused primarily on how the laboratory technician and the physician usually interpret a positive Lyme disease test. The other side of this diagnostic coin, of course, is a negative test. The controversy about seronegative disease was considered above. In the absence of more compelling evidence to the contrary, I accept the traditional view. That is, when Lyme disease is unlikely, and the test is being run as a screening test, then a negative test almost always means that the person does not have Lyme disease. We would say that under these conditions a negative test result is highly predictive.

But how is a negative test to be interpreted when the physician thinks that Lyme disease is likely—when there is a pre-test possibility of 50 percent, for example? With a test sensitivity of 96 percent, the chance that someone who actually has Lyme disease in this situation will have a negative test is 4 percent; on average, that means that one of twenty-five patients who really has *B. burgdorferi* infection will have a negative ELISA test. What does this mean for the person who is that one in twenty-five?

The encouraging news is that most experienced physicians will consider the possible explanations for a negative test when the history and physical exam suggest Lyme disease. One of the most common reasons for a negative ELISA test is that the blood sample was drawn before the antibodies in the blood reached a level high enough to be detected. During the first few weeks of infection, the antibody test, even for IgM antibody, may be negative. Antibodies generally reach detectable levels only after three to six weeks of infection. The IgM antibody test described above reduces this period to as little as one to two weeks, but then again this is at the cost of more false positives.

Another undisputed cause for a false-negative test is prior treatment with antibiotics during the first one to two weeks of disease. If antibiotics are begun early in the infection, typically when the skin rash first appears, the patient may never show a positive blood test. If antibodies are formed, they are formed at levels below the limit of detection by the test. Under these circumstances a negative test at some later time usually is of no consequence. Indeed, it probably means that the patient has been successfully treated.

In rare instances, however, the antibody test remains negative because of the early antibiotic treatment, but the infection goes on. It is as if the antibiotics prevent the body from making a good antibody response but are ineffective on their own at curing the disease. The worst possible diagnostic situation has occurred: the person is infected, but tests do not reveal the infection. An important clue to this uncommon phenomenon is the previous appearance in the patient of the erythema migrans skin rash, and treatment for this or some other early manifestation of infection. If the antibiotic was not prescribed—or taken—in the correct dosage, or for long enough, the infection may have been inadequately treated. Sometimes the problem is that the wrong antibiotic has been prescribed.

What can be done in a situation in which chronic Lyme disease is suspected by the physician, but the antibody test is negative on at least two occasions? Suppose, too, that in this situation there is no convincing history or medical documentation of the telltale erythema migrans rash. Again, most experts believe that this circumstance is uncommon. In this situation, there are at least three possible courses of action. The first is to treat the patient. The second is to perform the polymerase chain reaction assay or urine antigen assay (see below), tests that are promising but are not widely available and are still considered experimental. And the third is to test another part of the immune system besides antibodies. This involves examining a specific type of white blood cell, the *T lymphocytes.*

T lymphocytes, or "T cells," have become more common in daily discourse because of their significance in the course of disease in people with HIV infection. The fundamental problem for people with AIDS is that they have low numbers of one type of T cells; because of this deficiency of T cells, they are more susceptible to a variety of infections. T cells are an important aspect of the body's defense against invading microorganisms as well as against cancer. Just as there are antibodies that are uniquely directed against one type of microorganism, there are specialized T cells that are selective in what they recognize. The numbers of a particular kind of T cell increase substantially upon exposure to the microorganism in question. Accordingly, if there are antibodies directed against *B. burgdorferi* parts, then it is reasonable to think that there may also be specialized T cells that are specifically directed against something in or on these spirochetes. If the ELISA and Western blot tests can be used to detect the antibodies, then another test may be used to detect the specialized T cells. And, in fact, the blood and other body fluids of many Lyme disease patients have been found to contain T lymphocytes that are uniquely reactive with *B. burgdorferi.*

The test derived from these findings is called the *lymphocyte proliferation test.* In this test, white blood cells from the patient are exposed to parts of *B. burgdorferi,* and the response of the cells is measured in terms of their metabolic activity. If the cells become very active, that is an indication that T cells in the person's body recognize *B. burgdorferi*. The concept of this test did not originate with, and is not unique to, Lyme disease: there are other infections in which specific T cells can be assayed.

But whether the test is done to diagnose Lyme disease or to diagnose other infections, it can never be considered routine, since it is much more complex and costly to perform than most antibody tests. Few laboratories offer the test, and those that do usually offer it only on a research basis. False-positive reactions can also occur with T cell tests, as they do with the antibody tests. Still, for the person who appears to have Lyme disease but has had more than one negative antibody test, a positive lymphocyte proliferation test may be the only laboratory evidence of infection with *B. burgdorferi*.

Direct Detection: The "Gold Standard" for Diagnosis

Given the drawbacks of the antibody tests and the cost and relative unavailability of the lymphocyte proliferation test, we might well ask whether there are more direct and accurate ways to make a laboratory diagnosis of *B. burgdorferi* infection. There are, but they have their own problems. For most suspected cases of Lyme disease, the antibody test has the most to offer and is the least expensive assay. Still, increasingly there is a place for *direct testing* in the diagnostic process for Lyme disease. By direct testing we mean that the microorganism itself or part of the microorganism is identified in the patient. The advantage of a direct test is that, theoretically at least, there is less chance of a false-positive reaction.

Of all possible laboratory results, the least ambiguous is the growing of *B. burgdorferi* from a sample taken from the patient. This is the "gold standard" by which other tests are judged. In most patients with early Lyme disease the spirochetes can be cultured out of a snippet of skin taken from an erythema migrans skin rash. Such a skin biopsy is routinely performed for the diagnosis of other skin conditions, and the biopsy procedure can be done in a few minutes in the physician's office. Unfortunately, the next step—the cultivation of spirochetes from the biopsy—is less easy to perform. Few laboratories are equipped to culture *B. burgdorferi,* and even those that can may take two weeks to produce results. These spirochetes grow very slowly in the laboratory's culture medium as well as in the body. Another factor affecting how often the test is used is that the medium in which the spirochete grows has many components and is expensive.

Another option for the biopsy specimen is examination under the microscope. Skin biopsied for other reasons, such as suspected cancer, is usually handled in this way. Although this type of examination can reveal inflammation of the skin, by itself the picture is not diagnostic of Lyme disease. The same caveat applies to examination of other tissues, such as a nerve or the soft tissue in an affected joint. Spirochetes have to be seen in the microscope for the diagnosis to be confirmed. A problem for this type and most other types of direct testing is the scarcity of spirochetes in tissues, even those prominently involved, such as the skin or the joints. The procedure for revealing spirochetes differs from more commonly used procedures in the laboratory, and not every pathologist or technician is adept at using this technique.

Still, these deficiencies by themselves do not explain why the skin biopsy is not performed more often. After all, if there is a sure method to confirm the diagnosis, then growing or visually identifying the spirochete is that method. The demand for the procedure must not be there. If the demand were greater, more laboratories would offer cultivation of the spirochete and the special procedure for the microscopic exam. The principal reason that skin biopsies are seldom obtained for diagnosis is that the best chance for successful culture is when there is erythema migrans—and that is the circumstance in which a laboratory confirmation is least needed. A skin biopsy for diagnosis would only be indicated when the skin rash is atypical for Lyme disease or when a rash resembling erythema migrans occurs in a person in a geographic area not previously known to have Lyme disease.

Other body fluids suitable for sampling include, besides blood, the fluids that surround the brain and those that bathe the joints. The former is called *cerebrospinal fluid,* or CSF for short. The latter is called *synovial fluid.* The synovium is the tissue lining the cartilage and bones in the joints. Either the CSF or the synovial fluid is often examined in any case, if there is any sign of disease in either the brain or a joint. The presence of increased numbers of white blood cells and increased amounts of proteins in those fluids would be an indication of inflammation. However, cultivation of spirochetes from these locations is usually not successful, even if the diagnosis of Lyme disease is definite. The same applies to the examination and culture of tissues such as the synovium or the heart muscle. (A bit of heart muscle can be obtained with a tube snaked through the large veins into the heart.) Outside of a skin biopsy, the best source of a spirochete for culture is blood taken during the first two or three weeks of the infection (recall that *antibodies* to the spirochete, by contrast, seldom reach detectable levels until three to six weeks after infection starts). Once *B. burgdorferi* removes itself to the tissues, it seldom circulates in the blood.

Promising but Unproven Laboratory Tests

That spirochetes are occasionally discovered in cultures of the blood, cerebrospinal fluid, synovium, and heart of people with Lyme disease demonstrates that the microorganisms are there. What makes successful cultivation so difficult is that they are present in these locations only in very small quantities. A revolutionary technique offers a solution to this problem. If there are not enough organisms in the sample to begin with, this technique increases the number of bits of the spirochetes by up to a billionfold. The technique is the *polymerase chain reaction*, or PCR test.

Of course, only by actually growing the microorganism in culture can the numbers of whole cells be increased to this extent. What PCR testing does is circumvent the need for the organism itself to multiply. PCR accomplishes this—and within hours instead of days—by taking part of the DNA, the molecules of the cell's genes, and making millions of copies of it. If only a few spirochetes, or even just one, are present in the sample, this is sufficient for PCR to do its work. The multiplication, or amplification, of the DNA is achieved in a test tube by an enzyme that copies a piece of DNA over and over again. The process continues until the DNA can be easily detected in the laboratory. By starting with material for the amplification reaction which is unique to the microorganism in question, the accuracy of PCR testing is assured.

The advantage of the PCR test for Lyme disease is that traces of *B. burgdorferi* can be detected in samples that are seldom positive by culture. This was demonstrated by culturing the synovium and synovial fluid of patients with arthritis due to Lyme disease. There is also evidence that PCR can be used to detect the spirochete's DNA in the CSF and even in the urine. The significance of these findings is that a direct test for *B. burgdorferi* can now be done in late or chronic disease. PCR could also potentially be used to diagnose early Lyme disease by examining blood or skin samples.

Unfortunately, there is a downside to the PCR test: the procedure is almost too good for what it tries to do. PCR is very sensitive to contamination by stray DNA molecules in the laboratory. And with billions to trillions of copies of the DNA being made during the PCR process, it is not surprising that some of the DNA molecules get into the laboratory environment. They may land on bench tops, light fixtures, and walls, and they may float around on dust particles. One molecule dropping into the test tube is enough to invalidate the test. The risk of specimen contamination is so high that few laboratories are properly equipped and qualified to carry out the test for diagnostic purposes. The consequence of DNA contamination of the specimens is a false-positive test: someone may be inaccurately labeled as having Lyme disease as a result.

At present, PCR still has to be considered an experimental procedure. Any laboratory that offers the PCR test for Lyme disease diagnosis on a commercial basis probably also cautions that the test is being used "for research purposes" only. If the physician and the patient request PCR testing, the laboratory doing the test should be willing to provide information about their PCR test's accuracy. It is also reasonable to expect that the performance of the laboratory's test has been impartially evaluated by an outside agency. This applies to other nonstandardized tests, as well.

One of these other nonstandardized Lyme disease tests is the *urine antigen assay*. This direct test is based on the work of some researchers who found evidence of B. *burgdorferi* proteins, or antigens, in the urine of experimental animals and some patients. One inherent problem with this test is that it depends on antibodies to detect the antigens. The same types of cross-reactions that plague the antibody tests can occur in this situation. In the version of the test that was made widely available there was an unacceptably high number of false-positive reactions. A urine antigen assay currently offered by a laboratory in California sometimes must be performed on several samples from a patient before a "positive" is discovered. In other cases the test has been reported positive only after the patient was started on antibiotics. While further technical modifications may improve the accuracy of the urine antigen test, it is likely that a successful PCR test of urine will make such a test superfluous.

Future Expectations for Laboratory Testing

If all or most laboratories did the ELISA and Western blot tests the same way, with essentially the same reagents, and with the same sets of control sera, there is little doubt that the testing situation would be improved. Even though the pitfalls and problems inherent to the antibody test itself would remain, at least results obtained in one laboratory could be more easily compared with results obtained in another laboratory. And there would probably be better agreement across the country about just what a positive test is. Under these conditions, physicians and patients would not be faced by such a bewildering array of options.

At the present time there is a cottage industry of Lyme disease tests in the United States and some other countries. Most of the ELISA, IFA, and Western blot kits sold in the United States and in many other countries are produced by comparatively small companies. The reasons for this situation are many. One is the absence, early on, of leadership by federal agencies that had in the past provided nationwide standards for testing for emerging infectious diseases. A second reason was the hesitancy of large companies that make diagnostic tests to offer a Lyme disease test.

Standardization of the ELISA and Western blot assays is at last under way. In the future the accuracy and reliability of the procedures in laboratories will be evaluated more often by outside agencies than at present. One—perhaps the only—salutary aspect of our cottage industry situation is that the multiple variations of the ELISA and Western blot tests are competing against each other in the standardization and quality control process, and out of this competition the most accurate, the most predictive, test may emerge.

The combination of increased standardization and more universal quality control will also likely come to other areas of Lyme disease testing, especially the promising PCR tests of blood, body fluids, tissue, and urine. PCR tests are increasingly used in the laboratory diagnosis of many other types of diseases as well as in prenatal genetic screening, paternity cases, and criminal investigations. Further improvements in other PCR applications will likely benefit PCR testing for Lyme disease. There are still many remaining hurdles and challenges for laboratory diagnoses based upon PCR and related technologies, but the long-term future looks bright.

One of the possible ways of improving the inherent accuracy of the ELISA test is elimination of proteins and other spirochete parts that are cross-reactive. These are the parts that contribute to the comparatively high number of false-positive reactions in the ELISA test. The elimination could be achieved either by removing the cross-reactive parts from test material or by mixing together as a "cocktail" those proteins that have been found to be specific for *B. burgdorferi*. Now that several of these and other proteins have been cloned through genetic engineering, the latter approach becomes feasible.

Current Recommendations

There is optimism for the future, but what about the present? Many experienced and currently disgruntled physicians view the available Lyme tests as not being worth the trouble. In fact, in some states the numbers of Lyme disease tests ordered have decreased. After their initial enthusiasm about finally having a blood test for this condition, many physicians are now unsure how to interpret a positive or a negative test. These physicians may have treated patients who had positive test results but did not get better when treated with antibiotics. Or they may have seen patients who appeared to have Lyme disease but whose blood test results were negative. In my view, discouraging the use of laboratory testing would be like throwing the baby out with the bathwater. I believe that there is a place for blood assays and other tests in the diagnosis of Lyme disease. But a degree of healthy skepticism, as exemplified by the comments in this chapter, is recommended. With that we can address common questions about Lyme disease tests.

Who should have a blood test for Lyme disease? Anyone who has symptoms of Lyme disease and has been exposed to ticks in an area known to have Lyme disease transmission. (The currently recognized areas are described in Chapter 2.) Having visited or lived in a Lyme disease area within a reasonable time period—up to a year—of the start of symptoms is enough; that is, the person need not be aware of having had an actual tick bite or even remember seeing ticks. As discussed, many of the symptoms of late or chronic Lyme disease can be confused with other conditions, so the history of exposure becomes very important. If all the people with symptoms but without a history of exposure were tested, the majority of the positive results would be false positive.

What if the ELISA test is positive, "borderline," or "indeterminate"? In that case a Western blot assay should be performed. Usually this will be an IgG Western blot, but if the infection is in its first weeks, the IgM blot is also appropriate. In experienced hands and performed according to accepted standards, the combination of an ELISA with a follow-up Western blot is the most accurate test for antibodies to *B. burgdorferi.* That is, if the Western blot results are negative, there is little chance that the disease is caused by *B. burgdorferi.* However, if the Western blot results are positive, the patient's disease may still be caused by something else. Remember, the antibody test may also reveal past but inactive infection with *B. burgdorferi.*

What if the antibody test is negative? In almost all cases, except in early infections, this means that a *B. burgdorferi* infection is not ongoing. In a few rare cases of true Lyme disease, a negative blood test may be obtained. If a false-negative result is suspected, the next step is to repeat the test, perhaps at a different laboratory. If that second test is negative and Lyme disease is still strongly suspected, a choice must be made between watchful waiting, antibiotic treatment, and seeking out one of the more specialized and experimental tests described above.

If active Lyme disease is suspected and first the ELISA and then the Western blot results are positive, treatment is started. That is the subject of the next two chapters.

Antibiotic Treatment:
The Basics

■ Julia's rash almost surely was evidence of Lyme disease, the pediatrician decided. Treatment could start that day. But Julia's clinic chart showed that she had developed hives after taking penicillin two years earlier. Penicillin or related antibiotics, such as amoxicillin, were probably not a safe choice for her, then. Instead, she was given a prescription for doxycycline, from the tetracycline class of antibiotics. Julia was now old enough to be given a tetracycline. Her mother picked up the prescription, and Julia started the pills, to be taken twice daily, that afternoon. The next evening Julia told her mother that the rash on her leg and back itched and that she felt chilly. Her temperature was up to 101°F, and the rashes were redder. Her worried mother called the pediatrician, who reassured her that sometimes this happened after antibiotics were started. In fact, it was a sign, the physician said, that the diagnosis of Lyme disease had been correct. The physician again cautioned Julia to be sure to apply sunscreen if she was going to be in the sunlight for more than a few minutes, because the tetracyclines make people sensitive to the sun.

■ Werner was relieved to learn that his pain and muscle weakness were treatable and that they were not symptoms of something more serious, such as multiple sclerosis or a brain tumor. He was started on high doses of penicillin given intravenously—by vein. The penicillin was administered six times a day while he was in the hospital. After a week Werner's headache was less severe, and he was anxious to go home. The physicians switched his therapy to cefotaxime, which was given to him intravenously just twice a day. After being discharged from the hospital, Werner went in the morning and the evening to the outpatient clinic, where a nurse connected tubing to the needle in his arm and dripped in the antibiotic over a half hour. Between clinic visits Werner had to take care not to accidentally dislodge the needle in his arm and to make sure the site around the needle did not get dirty. But taking those extra precautions was certainly preferable to being in the hospital.

■ Catherine was treated for Lyme arthritis for four weeks with the antibiotic amoxicillin taken by mouth three times a day. She took a pill with water or juice when she first got up, another an hour or two after lunch, and one before retiring at night. During the first and second weeks of therapy the only problems were remembering to take the pills—especially the midday dose—and a few days of loose and more frequent bowel movements. At the end of the third week of treatment she noted several small red spots, first on her legs and then on her trunk and arms. The rash on her legs was the worst; many of the spots had grown together and turned a purplish red color. When Catherine reported the rash to her physician, she was advised to stop taking the amoxicillin and to begin taking cefuroxime (Ceftin). When she had the prescription for cefuroxime filled, Catherine found out that it was a more expensive antibiotic than the amoxicillin; but it only needed to be taken twice a day. Over the next few days Catherine's rash faded, and she finished her four weeks of antibiotic treatment without further incident.

■ Roy spent more than two weeks in the hospital. Once the diagnosis of Lyme disease of the heart had been made, his physicians began treating him with the antibiotic ceftriaxone (Rocephin) intravenously. After leaving the cardiac care unit, Roy spent several days in a heart ward where his heart rate could still be constantly monitored. Finally, his heart started beating at its normal rate and in its normal rhythm, and the cardiologist and infectious disease specialist decided that it was safe to remove the wire connecting the artificial pacemaker to Roy's heart. Roy developed gall bladder problems from the ceftriaxone during the second week, but he did not need surgery. He finished his therapy by receiving a second antibiotic, cefotaxime, intravenously. By that time he was on the regular ward of the hospital.

Are the experiences of Julia, Werner, Catherine, and Roy typical of people treated for Lyme disease? No. For one thing, two of these four people were hospitalized. Most people with Lyme disease are treated as outpatients—that is, at home. Overall, most people have fewer problems than the experiences of these four would suggest. Most patients have no side effects or only mild ones and do not have to switch antibiotics midcourse. Nevertheless, these stories demonstrate some of the inconveniences and complications of antibiotic therapy for Lyme disease. If the good news is that antibiotics usually help people with active *Borrelia burgdorferi* infections (see Chapter 7), the bad news is that there is sometimes a price (and not just a monetary price) to be paid for antibiotic therapy. And sometimes, as we'll see in this chapter, antibiotics fail. Finally, like other medicines, antibiotics can have beneficial effects in people which could not have been predicted.

How Antibiotics Work

An antibiotic is a chemical that is produced by one living organism and kills or otherwise inhibits another type of organism. One antibiotic was discovered when it was noted that bacteria were not growing around a mold originally isolated from an old cantaloupe. A clear, circular zone without any bacteria surrounded the mold. The mold produced a substance, penicillin, that stopped the bacteria in their tracks as they advanced toward it in a Petri dish. There are other types of antibiotics produced by molds, other fungi, and even bacteria. We usually think of antibiotics in terms of their use against bacterial infections, but some of the oldest and most common antibiotics have been used to treat cancer. These latter antibiotics work by killing tumor cells faster than they damage normal, healthy cells. With rare exceptions, antibiotics routinely used against bacteria are not effective against viruses, fungi, or parasites.

A broader definition of antibiotics includes chemicals created in the laboratory. Sulfa is such a drug and has actually been in use longer than penicillin. Most of the newer antibiotics are either completely synthesized in factories or are greatly modified versions of an antibiotic originally produced by a living organism.

By either definition, antibiotics menace bacteria, and in several ways. Some, such as penicillin, amoxicillin, and ceftriaxone, prevent the bacterium from constructing a sturdy wall beneath or around itself. In all of nature only bacteria have cell walls of this structure, and thus these antibiotics are not likely to interfere with the growth of human or other animal cells. An attractive feature of the penicillin group of antibiotics is that they usually kill the bacteria outright. When the cell walls of the bacteria are weakened, the bacteria literally burst at the seams. The numbers of bacteria can drop a hundredfold, a thousandfold, or even a millionfold within the first day of treatment. A drawback of most antibiotics in this group is that they have this effect only when the bacterial cells are dividing. If the bacteria are alive but are not growing in the body, antibiotics such as penicillin and ceftriaxone may fail. This can be a significant factor with a slow-growing bacterium such as *B. burgdorferi.*

Other kinds of antibiotics do not kill bacteria directly. Instead, their primary action is to stop the bacteria's growth. One antibiotic with this type of action is doxycycline, the antibiotic used to cure Julia's infection. Doxycycline is one of the tetracycline group of antibiotics. Other examples of inhibitory antibiotics are erythromycin and azithromycin. All of these antibiotics inhibit bacteria by interfering with one or more important steps in the bacterial cell's life and growth. Some antibiotics in this category prevent the bacteria from making proteins; like any other living creature, a bacterium without protein synthesis cannot become bigger. Other antibiotics halt the production of DNA, the cell's blueprints; without new DNA, one bacterium cannot become two.

While antibiotics are preventing the numbers of bacteria from getting out of hand, the body of the patient is producing antibodies. That is, simply by stopping the growth of the invading microorganisms the antibiotics gain the body's defenses time to mobilize. Moreover, whatever bacteria are already present may be weakened by the antibiotic by the time certain types of white cells, known as *phagocytes,* begin to flood the infected area. (The Greek-derived *phago-* refers to the ability of these cells to "eat" bacteria, viruses, and parasites, as well as the body's own debris.) In a disabled state the bacteria are more easily ingested by the scavenging white cells. If the person has low numbers of phagocytes or poorly functioning ones, antibiotics that only inhibit bacteria may not be as effective as antibiotics that kill directly. This becomes an important consideration, for instance, for people with cancer who are undergoing chemotherapy and may have few or no phagocytes. For people with fully functional immune systems, however, there usually is no particular advantage to using a lethal rather than a merely inhibitory antibiotic. Fortunately, people with most types of immune deficiencies, including AIDS, do not appear to be at especially high risk of contracting Lyme disease.

What may be more important than killing ability for an antibiotic's success is whether the antibiotic is capable of reaching the places in the body where the bacteria are. An antibiotic may perform spectacularly in a test tube, wiping out the equivalent of all the world's population within a few hours. But if it cannot first arrive at and then move into the infected organ or tissue, then that antibiotic will fail.

Furthermore, every antibiotic only has an effect above a certain concentration. The antibiotic's concentration may be high enough in the blood to kill or inhibit the infecting bacteria, but in a tissue its level may fall short. An oral antibiotic, that is, one taken by mouth, has to get from the stomach or intestine into the blood and then find its way out of the blood into the infected tissue. An antibiotic given by vein at least does not have to contend with the rough-and-tumble intestinal tract, filled as it is with food, a harsh acid, and bile—not to mention other medications that may compete with the antibiotic for absorption into the blood.

An example of this point—and one relevant to Lyme disease—is infection of the brain. As long as *B. burgdorferi* has not yet reached the brain, which is probably true for early localized Lyme disease, then an antibiotic's ability to reach into the brain is of little practical concern. However, if it is suspected that the spirochetes have become residents of the brain, then this becomes an issue in treatment decisions. Some antibiotics are much better than others in penetrating into the brain and the cerebrospinal fluid, the CSF, around it.

Protecting the brain is a layer or membrane that is incredibly restrictive about what it lets through. Just as some hormones circulating in the blood cannot get past this barrier, some antibiotics also fail to pass. If there is a severe infection of the brain, with large numbers of white cells in the CSF, this barrier becomes leaky. Then the amount of the drug going into the brain increases, sometimes dramatically. But this is an uncommon situation in Lyme disease. Even with a comparatively effective antibiotic for brain infections, the antibiotic's concentration in the brain is lower than in the blood and the rest of the body. This has implications for the dosage of the antibiotic, as discussed below.

In addition to whether it kills or only inhibits a specific bacterium, and whether it can penetrate into the affected tissue, a third determinant of an antibiotic's success or failure is whether it gets inside a person's cells. Some bacteria live only outside of cells—in the blood or urine, or in the spaces between cells in tissues—and in this case it is not important whether or not the antibiotic can pass into the inside of cells. However, some bacteria, such as those that cause tuberculosis, can prosper just as well within cells as outside of them. And some bacteria, such as those that cause Rocky Mountain spotted fever, are only productive when they are located within cells. In these situations an antibiotic that cannot reach the cell's interior will fail.

To achieve cell entry, the antibiotic must cross the membrane that surrounds the cell and then move to the location in the cell where the bacteria are proliferating. The membrane is made up of fats, and so antibiotics that are more soluble in fat have a better chance of crossing the membrane than do antibiotics that are more soluble in water. Other antibiotics can pass through the small holes that dot the cell membranes. Generally, antibiotics in the penicillin group, which includes ceftriaxone, are not as effective at getting inside cells as are antibiotics in the tetracycline or erythromycin groups.

Is an antibiotic's ability to get into cells relevant to Lyme disease treatment? That depends on who you talk to. Spirochetes have been thought of as primarily extracellular rather than intracellular bacteria, but a *B. burgdorferi* organism may spend some of its life inside cells. After all, for these bacteria to leave the blood and go into tissues, they must pass through the cells that line the blood vessels. But it does not take them long to make this passage through the cell's interior. The controversy is over whether a certain, probably small, number of these spirochetes can actually persist inside of cells for long periods of time. Some researchers think that they can, and believe that this persistence partly explains the occasional failures of antibiotic therapy. Their reasoning is that these intracellular spirochetes can escape the effects of the antibiotics that do not penetrate into cells well. When an antibiotic of that class is stopped, so the argument goes, the live bacteria inside the cells could reseed the rest of the body. There are many researchers who disagree; they don't believe that the occasional live spirochetes within cells are of much significance for treatment.

More research will resolve questions about the fate of *B. burgdorferi* in the body. Until then, clues will come from the successes and failures of different antibiotics used in the treatment of Lyme disease. If persistence of *B. burgdorferi* inside some of a person's cells is common, then antibiotics that reach killing or inhibitory levels inside of cells would be expected to be more effective than those that do not. So far, antibiotics such as penicillin and amoxicillin, which are not particularly good at getting into cells, appear to be as effective as those, like doxycycline, which are superior in this one respect.

Choosing an Antibiotic

Julia, Werner, Catherine, and Roy were treated with doxycycline, penicillin, cefotaxime, cefuroxime, amoxicillin, or ceftriaxone. Out of the hundred or so antibiotics that are now available, why did their physicians choose these particular drugs? The answer begins in the research laboratory and the medical library, includes the experiences of physicians and patients, and ends in the clinical trial, the one-on-one test of antibiotics.

There are several ways to match an antibiotic with a given infection. It might be done in trial-and-error fashion, by treating sick patients with various antibiotics and observing the outcomes; but this method could take months or years to come up with the correct match. (And a large number of people might become sicker or die in the process of eliminating useless medicines in this way.) An easier and safer—but not infallible—way to determine whether a specific antibiotic is effective in treating a specific infection is to test the drug against various bacteria in the laboratory. This is done by putting various amounts of the antibiotic of interest in culture tubes or in Petri plates and then seeing whether the bacteria are inhibited in their growth over the next few days. Antibiotics are restricted to a greater or lesser extent in the types of bacteria they combat. Such laboratory evaluations of new antibiotics reveal their strengths and weaknesses.

One antibiotic may be very effective against, say, the streptococcus, a cause of serious skin infections and sore throats, but not against the most common agents of bladder infections. Another antibiotic may have the opposite activity: good for urinary tract infections but not against "strep." Some antibiotics that were effective against many types of bacteria when they were first introduced into medical care now are limited in what they can do. This is the consequence of the ongoing evolution of bacteria to new forms that are said to be resistant to one or more antibiotics—that is, the new strains of the bacteria are not affected by the antibiotic in the way that their ancestors were. Resistance to an antibiotic usually occurs in one of two basic ways. The first is through a change in the enzyme or protein target for the antibiotic. If the antibiotic were a bolt and the bacterial protein the nut, one could say that in a resistant cell the nut has been changed, and the bolt no longer fits. The second way in which bacteria become resistant is by mounting a chemical counterattack that destroys the antibiotic.

Under the selective pressure of antibiotics in the hospital and community environment, the resistant "mutants" proliferate and spread from person to person. What happened to penicillin is a good example of how the development of resistant bacteria limits an antibiotic's usefulness. This one-time miracle drug used to be a lifesaving treatment against the staphylococcus, which causes boils in the skin and serious blood infections. But now most staphylococcus bacteria grow with impunity in the presence of formerly lethal amounts of penicillin. They produce an enzyme that breaks down the drug. By modifying the basic penicillin core—subtracting one chemical part and adding another—researchers produced new antibiotics that kill these penicillin-resistant staphylococcus bacteria and are not destroyed by the staphylococcus enzyme. Yet even as scientists were making these new antibiotics, there were among the hordes of bacteria—trillions of times more numerous than people on the earth—some organisms that were already resistant even to that next generation of drugs. Now these new mutants are common in hospitals, and the never-ending search for new antibiotics effective against them goes on.

Given this situation, an obvious goal of many pharmaceutical companies is to develop antibiotics that are effective against the widest possible variety of bacteria, including those that are now resistant to the older antibiotics. Such an antibiotic is prescribed often, because physicians feel safe using it even when they do not know what is causing the disease. When physicians prescribe medication without knowing what really is causing the disease, this is called "treating empirically." This approach is more common among physicians than is generally realized by patients and their families. In contrast, if an antibiotic works against a more restricted list of bacteria, then the physician is obliged to find out the actual cause of an infection before using that drug alone. Even if the cause of the infection becomes known, the bacteria may be resistant to the usual antibiotics. If the physician guesses incorrectly in picking an antibiotic, the disease goes unchecked.

The History of Lyme Disease Treatment

The history of Lyme disease shows that the path to choosing antibiotics for an infectious disease may not be the straightaway that I have described. That is, it may not be as simple as taking an infectious organism, checking different antibiotics against it, and then using the effective ones to treat patients. In the case of Lyme disease, an effective antibiotic treatment was used three decades before anyone knew what caused the disease—before there was any microorganism to test in the laboratory.

Some physicians in Europe had the hunch that erythema migrans was an infectious disease. They knew that the disease was carried by ticks. This was evidence that an infectious agent was involved, but what kind was unknown. Ticks were known to carry infectious viruses, one-celled animals, worms, and various kinds of bacteria. If a bacterium from a tick was causing the skin rash, there was a chance that an antibiotic would work. Conversely, an antibiotic would not be expected to work against viruses or most protozoa. Since there were few antibiotics available in the 1950s, choosing between them was not as difficult as it would be today. Two of the possibilities were penicillin and tetracycline. Using these antibiotics, physicians in different parts of Europe found that they were effective for erythema migrans.

When Lyme disease was discovered in the United States, the connection with erythema migrans in Europe was not yet apparent. The first group of patients in Lyme, Connecticut, were notable for their joint problems, not their skin rashes. An infectious disease was likely, but some type of virus headed the list of suspects, and so antibiotics were not used. As more cases of Lyme arthritis accumulated, though, Allen Steere and his colleagues found out that many of the patients recalled having had a skin rash before the arthritis or nerve disorder appeared. When they saw the rash, the similarity of Lyme disease in the United States to the erythema migrans disease reported in Europe was clear. Patients in the United States were then treated with penicillin, with good effect. Those who received the antibiotic had shorter durations of illness and were less likely to develop arthritis than were those who were not so treated.

The cause of Lyme disease was identified as a spirochete in the early 1980s. Other spirochetes, such as those that cause syphilis, were known to be susceptible to penicillin and tetracycline, so the success of these antibiotics in treating Lyme disease in its North American and European forms made sense. The newly discovered *B. burgdorferi* organism was subsequently examined in the laboratory and confirmed to be susceptible to penicillins and tetracyclines.

The Lyme disease bacterium was also killed or inhibited in laboratory tests by chloramphenicol, erythromycin-type antibiotics known as macrolides, and cephalosporins. Cephalosporins are similar enough to penicillins to be chemical cousins. Ceftriaxone, cefotaxime, and cefuroxime are cephalosporins commonly used to treat Lyme disease. The macrolides in use now are erythromycin, azithromycin, and clarithromycin. Chloramphenicol is an older antibiotic of a different class and structure. It is particularly good at getting into the brain and inside of cells, but in rare circumstances it has a deadly side effect.

Several other antibiotics fell short in the inhibiting and killing tests performed in the laboratory, although, luckily, there were no strains of the Lyme disease spirochete that had the type of rapidly spreading antibiotic resistance described above. The less effective antibiotics included sulfa drugs and ciprofloxacin and related antibiotics. Still, researchers wondered whether these antibiotics might possibly be effective in an animal or a person despite their failure or unimpressive performance in a test tube. Might physicians be missing opportunities with some antibiotics because the test tube results are misleading? This is possible, but chances are slim that the lab results are unduly pessimistic. It's more likely that an antibiotic that succeeds in the laboratory will perform disappointingly in people. Using a drug that fails in the laboratory will not be of benefit in the treatment of Lyme disease. Indeed, if such antibiotics are associated with improvement in a patient's condition, this is probably not because the antibiotic was surprisingly effective against Lyme disease: the improvement may have been coincidence; the antibiotic may have had a placebo effect; the original diagnosis of Lyme disease may have been wrong; or the beneficial effects of the drug may have been non-specific—that is, not associated with the killing of bacteria.

Erythromycin has not really been a failure as a treatment, but it did not live up to the expectations created by its performance in the laboratory, where in small amounts it stopped spirochete growth. Studies first in experimental animals and then in people with Lyme disease showed that erythromycin was less effective in live animals and people than were some antibiotics that performed less dazzlingly in the laboratory. Vancomycin is another antibiotic that worked well in the test tube but not in experimental animals.

The effectiveness of erythromycin and other drugs is often studied by means of controlled clinical trials. In a controlled clinical trial, some patients are given the medication that is being tested, and other patients are given either another medication, one already proven to work, or a placebo, such as a disguised sugar pill. Which patients receive which pill is determined randomly, and is kept a secret. The best trials are "blinded" in the sense that neither the physicians nor the people in their care know which type of pill is given to each individual. The truth about who got what is revealed only at the end of the study. Allowing neither patient nor physician to know who is taking what minimizes the risk that a conscious or unconscious bias will affect the outcome of the drug trial.

The first controlled, blinded trial of antibiotic treatment for Lyme disease was done at a time when there was no convincing evidence that antibiotics would work at all for this condition. Consequently, some of the patients in this first study did not get any antibiotic. They were injected with a salt solution instead of penicillin. In such a situation, when the efficacy of any treatment is questioned, it is ethical for some patients not to be treated. After all, it is conceivable that the therapy will cause more harm than the lack of treatment. Antibiotics are not without side effects or cost. As it happened, the people who took antibiotics in that first study of antibiotic treatment of Lyme disease did do better than those who did not take antibiotics. And since that first study, patients in all clinical trials for Lyme disease have gotten some form of antibiotic.

One would think that by now—almost two decades after the first antibiotic trial—many such studies would have been conducted comparing the effectiveness of different antibiotics in the treatment of Lyme disease, or comparing different dosages and durations of treatment with particular antibiotics. Regrettably, however, the clinical trials for Lyme disease treatment have been comparatively limited. Many of the trials that have been carried out have involved small numbers of patients or have been restricted in the number of variables examined. Valuable lessons came from these studies, but there remain several questions that can only be answered by a controlled trial. In many instances, treatment decisions are still empirical: the physician cannot provide compelling evidence one way or another about a course of action. The lack of information for physicians regarding treatment is especially frustrating, because chronic Lyme disease can be subtle enough that a clear-cut improvement or worsening of the condition may be difficult to discern. There is a tendency for this disease to wax and wane in severity on its own, so the physician and the patient must both wonder: When the illness wanes during or soon after treatment, is the improvement attributable to the antibiotic or to the natural course of the disease?

The Placebo Effect

Besides coincidence, there is another reason that giving credit to an antibiotic for a patient's improved condition might be undeserved: the placebo effect. Placebos—such as the salt solution in the example above—are used routinely in clinical trials. But when a placebo is used in practice it has come to mean something more sinister.

In common usage the word *placebo* has a negative connotation, being associated with both underhandedness and ineffectiveness. Not that many years ago, though, physicians knowingly or innocently depended on the placebo effect in treating most of the diseases they confronted. This was because for much of medicine's history there were only a handful of drugs that had specific, identified actions. Now physicians have available to them hundreds of effective therapies for hundreds of diseases and conditions. It is understandable, then, that when a physician resorts to a placebo, this action is seen as somewhat dishonest, regardless of whether it was well intentioned or not.

Behind this scorn is the suspicion that placebos are used to fool people, that they are the tool of quacks and charlatans. But is that a fair assessment? Can't placebos actually help people? Obviously, physicians in the past thought so. Much of their living, after all, was made by prescribing placebos, and few physicians before the twentieth century were run out of town or tarred-and-feathered. Some argue now that many of the alternative treatments available through health food and vitamin stores are nothing more than placebos. That may or may not be so, but the fact is that placebos *do* work—at least in the sense that many patients benefit from them.

Numerous studies of the placebo effect have been carried out. In many of these the subjects got either nothing or a pill, sometimes an injection, which they thought would help them. In other studies the people received either no treatment, a placebo, or a medication that had been shown to truly relieve or improve the condition. Both the subjects receiving the placebo and those receiving the effective therapy were told that the treatment would help them. Under these trial conditions, when the placebo was compared with no treatment, the beneficial effects of the placebo were seen in roughly one-third of cases: 25 to 40 percent of the people getting the placebo perceived an improvement in their condition which was above and beyond that noted by subjects receiving nothing. The proportion of people who report a good effect from placebos is actually higher when the "therapy" is given intravenously or is some type of operation. In general, the more invasive and intensive the treatment, the greater is the placebo effect.

Most of these studies were done with chronic diseases, such as rheumatoid arthritis, but similar effects were also seen in more acute conditions, such as headache or pain after an operation. A placebo would not be used under conditions in which a medicine has a clear-cut beneficial effect, such as in cases of pneumonia, in which antibiotics are effective, or asthma attacks, which are treated with epinephrine. A placebo is not likely to stop the diarrhea of cholera, repair a fractured bone, or heal an inflamed appendix. Placebos have their greatest effect in the treatment of subjective symptoms such as pain, headache, insomnia, and fatigue.

The implication still may be that those people who respond to placebos are particularly suggestible or easily hoodwinked. One might also argue, circularly, that if someone receives benefit from a placebo, his or her degree of discomfort must not have been very great. In actuality, placebos have worked in situations in which the presence of pain is not in doubt, for instance, in patients after surgery. If people who respond to placebos are somehow different in their personalities or behavioral traits from those who do not, this is beside the point. The wonder is that the placebos work at all.

And how might they be working? The answer, still incomplete, would be beyond the scope of this book; indeed, an entire book could be devoted to the subject. Such a book would consider the increasing amount of information on what has been called, among other names, the mind-body interaction. What better example of the influence of the mind over bodily functions than the placebo effect? An individual's belief that a pill can lead to decreased pain or an increased sense of well-being is apparently of great consequence to the effectiveness of the pill, even if that pill is made of sugar. In that case it is not the pill itself, but the belief and hope, that matters. That hope may be fostered by the physician or other healer providing the placebo. A pill dispensed indifferently or with little outward expectation of success may not provide any relief, no matter what it is. The physician is a "drug" of a sort, too, and in this sense can be dispensed with skill and compassion or with clumsiness and insensitivity.

The scientific findings to date clearly show that placebos can produce relief of various types of symptoms, perhaps by a mechanism that works through the local and distant connections of the brain. There are, for example, naturally occurring chemicals in the brain that mimic the opiate pain relievers, such as morphine. It is possible that these so-called endorphins are released through the hope and optimism engendered by a placebo, providing one explanation of the temporary pain relief provided by the placebo effect.

Whether placebos, or more accurately, the belief or hope in the placebo, can lead to partial or complete reversal of the basic disease process is less certain. Stories abound of optimistic cancer patients surviving longer than their more despondent counterparts. This life-sustaining hope appears to spring from a deeper source than what might be packaged in the form of a pill, but more remains to be discovered about how placebos work, and especially about the long-term effects of this ancient medicine.

Unintended Effects of Antibiotics

A medicine may be effective in reducing symptoms because it stops the disease process or because it acts as a placebo. Accordingly, we would say that if an antibiotic benefited a patient with chronic Lyme disease, it was because the drug kept *B. burgdorferi* from growing and/or because the patient believed that it would help. A third possibility is that the antibiotic was irrelevant to the patient's improvement: the patient would have improved regardless of the treatment, placebo effect or no. There is a fourth possible explanation, one that has as yet less weighty scientific support: the antibiotic may have an effect on the body that is independent of its effect on *B. burgdorferi*.

These other actions of the antibiotic can be thought of as side effects. Side effects of antibiotics may be minor nuisances, they may be catastrophes, or they may be something in between. These negative side effects are considered in the rest of this chapter. But there are also "side effects" of antibiotics that may be thought of as beneficial, and we'll look at them first.

Dermatology is an area of medicine that perhaps more than others appreciates the direct effects of antibiotics on the body as well as on bacteria. This phenomenon has been noted in the treatment of acne, one of the most common "disorders" of humans. Theories of acne treatment were once based solely on the notion that antibiotics would inhibit certain skin bacteria from growing, thereby preventing pimples. Although to a certain extent these antibiotics do change the bacterial flora of the skin, perhaps a more significant action of the antibiotics is reduction of inflammation. Tetracycline and related antibiotics are one of the most frequently prescribed medicines for acne; teenagers may take tetracycline every day for months at a time. Not only can tetracyclines inhibit bacteria but they also have an anti-inflammatory action. Acne "spots" are little, isolated areas of swelling and white blood cells in the skin, and therefore, in treating acne, tetracycline may be more useful for its anti-inflammatory properties than for its antibacterial effects. Other antibiotics appear to have similar abilities to reduce inflammation.

Could tetracycline, doxycycline, and other antibiotics be having an anti-inflammatory action in patients thought to have chronic Lyme disease? An enigma is that some patients with symptoms compatible with but not diagnostic of Lyme disease feel better while on antibiotic therapy. What distresses them and their caregivers is the return of symptoms after what should have been an adequate length of treatment. Antibiotics are again started, with partial or complete improvement. They may be taken conscientiously for weeks or even months. But, in what is not an unusual story, the symptoms return sooner or later after the antibiotics are stopped.

There is controversy about whether this is Lyme disease or not. Some researchers and clinicians believe that the apparent ineffectiveness of antibiotics, even when given in large doses and for extended treatment schedules, is proof, by exclusion, that the illness is not Lyme disease. Their reasoning is that disease caused by living *B. burgdorferi* would have been cured by the lengthy course of antibiotics. Others look at the same findings and conclude instead that Lyme disease requires weeks, months, and sometimes years of treatment, and that even then the patient may not be cured. The best some patients may hope for, according to this more pessimistic view, is that the disease can be controlled. An alternative and still untested view of the same phenomenon is that antibiotics are having a beneficial effect in these patients, but that this effect is due to their anti-inflammatory rather than antibacterial actions. According to this explanation, whether the illness started as a *B. burgdorferi* infection or not is almost immaterial.

The Safety of Antibiotics

These salutary actions of antibiotics, whether intended or not, are complemented by a good overall safety record. Of all types of medications, antibacterial antibiotics are among the safest. This is true because of the aforementioned differences in the structures and metabolisms of bacterial and human cells. There is inherently less chance of toxicity with antibiotics than with medications that are supposed to work on human cells, tissues, organs, and systems.

The relative safety of antibiotics is one reason why physicians prescribe them frequently in the office and in the hospital. If an infection is suspected and antibiotics that inhibit a broad variety of bacteria are available, there is little perceived downside to dispensing an antibiotic. Certainly it is less risky to use an antibiotic than to use an anticancer drug or a powerful steroid. Anticancer drugs and steroids routinely, not exceptionally, have serious side effects, including suppression of the immune system, anemia, fragile skin, and loss of hair. Starting an anticancer drug is not a trivial decision; starting an antibiotic often seems to be. But antibiotics are not without risk, and possible deleterious effects should be taken into account in treatment decisions. There is, as they say, no free lunch, even with antibiotics, the prototypical "magic bullets."

In developing a new antibiotic, the first priority is to determine whether a candidate compound kills or inhibits bacteria; the first priority is not usually safety. Thousands of compounds with these activities have been discovered or produced. But most of these antibiotics now sit almost forgotten on the backroom shelves of pharmaceutical companies or research institutes. These antibiotics may have come on like gangbusters when killing bacteria in the test tube, but they were also, to their discoverer's or inventor's chagrin, poisonous to animals. This toxicity may have been discovered in studies of human or other animal cells growing in the laboratory. The cells may have grown poorly or died, or they may have showed other signs of distress. Some antibiotics proceed to animal testing before their less-than-benign properties are revealed. The treated animals may develop seizures or enlarged, sick livers as a result of the drug.

If the drug under consideration survives this gauntlet of laboratory and animal tests, the next step in the evaluation is a trial with human volunteers. These are often college or medical school students and are usually paid for their participation. The volunteers are given the antibiotic either by mouth, by injection into a muscle, or by injection directly into the blood. The purpose of these early tests in humans is not to see if the antibiotic works against infections—the animal tests are usually predictive of this. Instead, the principal aim is to pick up any signs that the drug is toxic to people. This is done by monitoring the volunteers by questionnaire for symptoms such as headache, nausea, and blurred vision; by physical exams for signs of disordered organ function, such as a skin rash or lack of coordination; and by blood and urine tests for abnormalities in the blood, liver, kidneys, glands, intestinal tract, and muscles.

If there are no abnormalities or a tolerable number of minor abnormalities after this stage of testing, the Food and Drug Administration—the FDA—customarily allows more extensive testing involving human volunteers. Additional people receive the drug in various strengths and for durations relevant to real-life therapeutic situations. Sometimes abnormalities become apparent only when larger groups of people are tested. These side effects may be fairly negligible, such as a mild nausea or headache, or they may be more worrisome, such as a declining number of white blood cells.

In the final stages of testing, the new antibiotic is tried out on patients in hospitals, clinics, or physicians' offices. These patients or their guardians are informed of the test and sign a consent form if they agree to participate. At this point the principal question is whether the drug works to cure the infection. But participating patients are also routinely monitored for side effects. Toxicity is still a concern. An unavoidable problem in using hospitalized patients for this stage of testing is that these people commonly have other diseases besides the infection. These coexisting conditions complicate interpretation of possible signs of antibiotic toxicity. Is the elevated liver chemical in the blood due to the patient's alcoholism, or to the new antibiotic? Is the skin rash from the new antibiotic, or from the other drug that was started the day before? Sometimes it is impossible to discriminate between these possibilities.

Although the evaluation process for a new antibiotic might be strenuous, it might not be flawless or infallible. The antibiotic might perform admirably on many counts at curing patients of their infections. Nevertheless, unforeseen side effects might be detected only after the drug has been approved for sale and even larger numbers of people have been treated. The frequency and magnitude of such effects may be tolerable, especially if patients given placebos in controlled clinical trials reported similar side effects. (Placebos are associated with the creation of new symptoms as well as with their relief.) However, some side effects may be serious enough that either the antibiotic is withdrawn from the market or caution in its use is urged. An example is chloramphenicol, which was one of the most effective antibiotics when it was first introduced four decades ago. But some patients treated with this drug developed life-threatening or fatal blood disorders. This was rare enough, and chloramphenicol was uniquely valuable enough for some infections, that there was little choice but to continue to use the antibiotic, albeit more cautiously and with greater discrimination. As equally effective or more effective antibiotics were introduced, the amount of chloramphenicol used in practice declined.

In the example of chloramphenicol, a new generation of safer antibiotics supplanted an older, more hazardous drug. As a rule, though, antibiotics long in use have the advantage that their side effects are a known quantity. After millions of people have been treated with penicillin or tetracycline, to name two older antibiotics, the appearance of hitherto unsuspected side effects is unlikely. The chances of any given effect occurring are predictable, and these risks can be weighed against the estimated benefits from the drug. In contrast, a newly introduced antibiotic, for all its touted and real benefits, may have yet to show its full range of side effects, which may become apparent after the drug is used more widely. For example, a new antibiotic called temafloxin was put on the market in January 1992 but was withdrawn from the market in June of that same year after several people taking it developed severe low blood sugar.

The Adverse Effects of Some Antibiotics

Ceftriaxone is one of the most commonly used antibiotics for the treatment of Lyme disease. After ceftriaxone had already been approved for use and had been introduced into the market, a disturbing association became more noticeable. About 2 percent of people taking the antibiotic for Lyme disease developed gall bladder disease. Although the gall bladder problems usually resolve after people stop taking the antibiotic, in many cases abdominal surgery for gall bladder removal is carried out. The risk of developing a side effect that could lead to costly, major surgery must be considered in making decisions about treatment.

Among Lyme disease antibiotics, ceftriaxone is not alone in having mild to severe side effects. A common side effect of most antibiotics is diarrhea or loose stools. This usually results from an ecological change, not in the outside environment but in the environment inside the person. A human is exposed to the rest of the world not just at the skin's surface but also in the intestinal and respiratory tracts, from the nose and mouth to the anus. The small and large intestine provide a particularly luxuriant and diversified environment.

If the skin is analogous to a desert in its variety of life, the intestine is like a rain forest. Contained within the elongated sac, twenty or so feet in length, are huge numbers of different types of bacteria and sometimes protozoa and worms. There are intestinal bacteria in humans and other animals that have yet to be named, because they cannot be grown outside of a person. There are also complex inter-actions between the bacteria, many types of which depend on others for their growth. Because of these complicated relationships, often involving three or more different types of bacteria, it is difficult to predict the effect of making even one alteration in the intestinal en-vironment. The consequences may be minimal, or they may be cat-astrophic.

Antibiotics often disrupt this inner environment. Even if only one type of intestinal bacterium is affected by the antibiotic, the change in its numbers may be enough to have many consequences for other bacteria. For instance, the elimination of one bacterial type may permit a second bacterium, whose numbers had been kept in check by the first, to thrive. In larger numbers the second bacterium may make enough toxins or other chemicals to cause diarrhea. In-frequently but dramatically, the resurgent bacterium causes severe diarrhea, cramps, and ulcers of the intestine. This condition can be life threatening, especially for infants and patients who are already infirm. One of the opportunistic bacteria causing severe diarrhea in some people taking antibiotics is called *Clostridium difficile*. There is a laboratory test for this bacterium and the toxin that it produces. Once this particular culprit has been identified, other antibiotics, usually either vancomycin or metronidazole taken by mouth, can be used to reduce the numbers of *C. difficile* in the intestine.

Another possible consequence of overgrowth of more deleterious microorganisms is a yeast infection of the vagina. *Candida* yeasts are a type of fungus and are not affected by most antibiotics. When bac-terial species in the vagina are killed off, the *Candida* organisms in-crease in numbers in the absence of competition and cause vaginal discharge and irritation.

The less severe forms of diarrhea sometimes are treated or pre-vented by consuming yogurt containing active cultures of the bacte-ria responsible for making this ancient derivative of milk what it is. Although this form of prophylaxis does not work in all instances, it probably won't do any harm, and it may help. The nausea that some antibiotics cause is usually a direct effect of the antibiotic on the stomach lining and muscles. Yogurt will not prevent this side effect, but often taking the antibiotic with meals helps reduce or eliminate the nausea.

Some antibiotics should not be taken during meals or close to mealtime because the presence of food in the stomach and intestine decreases absorption of the antibiotic into the blood. Tetracycline is an antibiotic that should not be taken within a hour before a meal or one to two hours after a meal. If tetracycline is to be taken four times a day, finding a good time to take a pill may prove difficult.

One of the other warnings given to people taking the tetracycline-type drugs is to avoid a lot of sun exposure: good advice at all times, but especially so with these antibiotics. Tetracyclines are noted for their tendency to increase a person's sensitivity to sunlight. They penetrate to the upper layers of the skin, and the chemical structure of the antibiotic is such that the effects of the sun's rays on the skin are magnified. The result may be a skin rash or severe sunburn in areas exposed to sunlight.

Some of the less common but sometimes serious side effects of antibiotics are impairment of kidney or liver function, a decrease in the number of blood cells, inflammation of the vein where the antibiotic is given, a tendency toward bleeding, intolerance of alcohol, diminished hearing, nerve damage, insomnia, and dizziness. Each type of antibiotic does not produce all of these effects: certain antibiotics are associated with certain side effects. For instance, dizziness is a much more likely side effect for someone taking the antibiotic minocycline than for someone taking other antibiotics of the tetracycline class.

Drug Interactions

Some side effects of antibiotics happen only when the antibiotics are taken along with other medications. There are so many of these so-called drug interactions that can occur that even experienced physicians, nurses, and pharmacists cannot keep all of them in mind. Most of the interactions are of little consequence, but some are more serious. Some people have developed a life-threatening disturbance of the heartbeat after taking macrolide antibiotics, such as erythromycin and azithromycin, along with the antihistamine terfenadine (better known as Seldane). Likewise, if a tetracycline and digitalis are being taken at the same time, the antibiotic may increase the toxicity of the heart drug.

A seemingly less consequential drug interaction is the effect of antacids, especially those with aluminum compounds, on the absorption of tetracycline. The antacid drug binds the tetracycline in the stomach and reduces the amount of antibiotic that can be absorbed from the intestine. Although this interaction does not produce a direct effect on a treated person, it could lead to a failure of the treatment of a disease such as Lyme disease, because not enough tetracycline is absorbed to inhibit the growth of the disease-causing organism.

As the number of medications increases, the possibilities for adverse interactions will also likely increase, probably geometrically. Computer programs have been created that will identify potential interactions, and there are several reference books that provide data on all known drug interactions. Your physician and your pharmacist have access to these materials and will almost certainly consult one of them if there are any questions about a potential interaction. You can expect, too, that they will ask you what medicines you're taking—the physician, so that he or she can make safe decisions about prescribing medications for you, and the pharmacist, so that he or she can caution you about drug interactions, or even call your physician to discuss the medications, if there's a potential for a problematic interaction. If you are not asked, you should be sure to report to your physician and pharmacist all of the medications that you are presently taking. It's not a bad idea to carry a list of your current medications with you, especially if you see different physicians for different medical problems.

Allergic Reactions

Some complications of Lyme disease therapy cannot be blamed solely on the antibiotics. In these cases it is the person's own immune system, and not the drug itself, that causes most of the damage. One such immune response is an allergic reaction to the antibiotic. Whether the person has Lyme disease or not is irrelevant, since an allergic reaction to this specific drug could just as easily happen during treatment of a strep throat or gonorrhea.

Such a reaction does not usually occur the first time someone is treated with an antibiotic; it may happen the second, third, fourth, or umpteenth time that the person takes that antibiotic or one that is chemically similar to it. Just as people are not born with an allergy to house dust or to flower pollen, people are not born with an allergy to penicillin. A substance such as these begins to produce allergic symptoms in a person only after he or she has been exposed to the substance and his or her body has produced lots of antibodies to it. By the next time the susceptible person is exposed to the substance, these antibodies have made the person supersensitive to it. When the person enters a dusty room, walks past a field of goldenrod, or swallows a penicillin tablet, there's trouble.

People who are allergic to airborne substances usually develop hay fever (sneezing, itchy nose, watery eyes) or asthma (labored breathing, chest constriction, coughing). A drug allergy shows up in a different way, similar to the way bee-sting sensitivity shows up. The most dangerous kind of drug allergy occurs suddenly, within minutes of receiving the drug through a vein or in a muscle or, less likely but possibly, after taking the drug orally. As with a severe bee-sting allergy, the patient's blood pressure drops and breathing becomes very difficult. If adrenaline is not administered soon after the start of this reaction, the patient may die. Fortunately, these overwhelming, potentially fatal reactions are rare; for example, severe reactions to penicillin occur about once in ten thousand injections of the drug.

A related but less severe reaction is hives or welts over the body. These typically appear within a few hours of being given the antibiotic. They are usually smooth in texture, raised above the skin, and slightly redder than the surrounding area, and are often itchy. Julia could not take amoxicillin because she had previously developed hives after taking penicillin, a chemically similar antibiotic.

A third type of allergic reaction is delayed in its appearance, occurring several days after the start of the antibiotic treatment. This reaction looks similar to the rash of measles. There are small, red, slightly raised spots, sometimes over the whole body and sometimes limited to certain areas, such as the legs. Between 1 and 5 percent of people taking an antibiotic develop a rash. A person who has such a reaction usually but not always has to stop taking the drug and, if treatment has not been completed, replace it with another. Catherine had a delayed reaction to amoxicillin.

That antibiotics can be lethal for some people means that they should not be prescribed indiscriminately—that is, without making every effort to determine whether the antibiotic under consideration might cause a problem for a particular individual. Before prescribing an antibiotic, the physician will ask the patient questions about any allergic reactions to medicines in the past. A patient's report of a possible allergic reaction to an antibiotic steers consideration away from that antibiotic and toward another. One problem in making this determination is that many people remember having had some sort of unpleasant symptoms after taking an antibiotic. But was this an allergic reaction or a side effect of the medication? If what is reported is nausea, diarrhea, minor dizziness, or headache, it's not likely that this was a true allergic reaction, and there is a low risk of sudden collapse from receiving the same antibiotic. An indication of serious trouble ahead is more likely when the patient tells a story of difficult breathing or a rash, particularly hives, occurring within a few minutes or hours of taking the pill or shot. Most reports of a measles-like, spotty red rash with an onset within days of starting an antibiotic are also taken as evidence of a drug allergy, even if a less serious one.

If there is any suspicion that the patient may be allergic to a specific antibiotic, then this drug or a closely related one should not be given. There are alternative antibiotics that would not be expected to produce an allergic reaction. For example, if the patient reports hives two days after receiving oral ampicillin, then not only ampicillin but also penicillin, amoxicillin, and other penicillin-type drugs should be avoided. A safer choice would be one of the tetracycline or macrolide drugs. This was the decision Julia's physician made after reading her medical chart. (The cephalosporin-type antibiotics, like cefuroxime, are related to penicillin but are different enough in structure that they can sometimes be used in someone who is allergic to penicillin. In this situation the risk of an allergic cross-reaction is low but not nonexistent.)

Occasionally the only choice left is to treat the patient with an antibiotic that he or she may be allergic to. This would be true, for example, if the person were hypersensitive to all the types of antibiotic that would be appropriate for treatment. Or perhaps after other antibiotics have failed the only reasonable alternative is the antibiotic that had on another occasion given the person a rash. In situations like this, the person can be "desensitized" to the drug through a gradual, incremental, and well-monitored series of exposures to it. The process is similar to that of giving allergy shots to people who are hypersensitive to specific foods or to environmental substances such as house dust. The difference is that antibiotic desensitization occurs over a course of a day instead of the several weeks to months involved in allergy shots.

The Jarisch-Herxheimer Reaction

After starting their antibiotics, a minority of patients with early Lyme disease become sicker instead of better. This happened to Julia. Within one or two days of beginning treatment, the rash of erythema migrans may become redder and slightly painful or itchy. The person's temperature usually rises one or two degrees Fahrenheit, and the person may have general achiness. But this apparent setback is neither an antibiotic side effect nor an allergic reaction.

Unlike an allergy or side effect, what has been called the Jarisch-Herxheimer reaction (after the two physicians who described it) occurs only when the person has been infected with a spirochete. The person could take the same antibiotic for another type of infection without suffering the same outcome. What happens in the Jarisch-Herxheimer reaction is that the antibiotic kills a large number of *B. burgdorferi* cells, and the person responds to these dead spirochetes by releasing cytokines and certain hormones. This local and systemic outpouring of body chemicals leads to increased inflammation at the erythema migrans site, elevates the temperature, and creates overall achiness. Thus, the Jarisch-Herxheimer reaction, while discomforting to the patient and to the physician first encountering it, is actually a sign that the antibiotics are working and that the diagnosis of Lyme disease is probably correct. Within a couple of days the symptoms of the reaction abate and general improvement follows.

Some patients and their physicians have reported similar but not identical reactions during the treatment of illnesses thought to be late Lyme disease. In these situations there is usually no fever or skin rash at the time treatment begins. The reaction these patients describe is an increase in the joint and muscle aches, a greater fatigue, and perhaps chilliness. Whether or not this is a true Jarisch-Herxheimer reaction is not clear at this time. A heightening of symptoms more than two days after the start of antibiotics is unlikely to be such a reaction. Moreover, these experiences are usually entirely subjective; in the absence of objective findings such as fever or worsening of the rash, a patient's report of increased aches and fatigue after starting antibiotics cannot be taken as evidence in favor of a diagnosis of chronic Lyme disease.

Some Antibiotic "Don'ts"

Antibiotics are generally safe, but under some conditions certain antibiotics should not be used at all and others should be used in reduced amounts. Pregnancy is one such condition. Care must be taken in the use of any medication, including antibiotics, during pregnancy. Among the older antibiotics, tetracycline and related drugs should not be prescribed for pregnant women. One reason is that pregnant women are more sensitive to the toxic effects of tetracycline. The other reason is that this class of antibiotics will stain the developing teeth of the fetus a brown or yellow color. The bones are also affected, though these effects would not be visible. Because of this effect, tetracyclines should also not be taken by women who are nursing and by children younger than nine, the age at which the permanent teeth have finished coming in.

Many newer antibiotics are also avoided during pregnancy, not so much because they are associated with known side effects on pregnant women or their babies as because the effects are not known at all. In trials for toxicity and effectiveness, antibiotics are not tested on pregnant women, primarily because of concerns of safety and fear of lawsuits. Although these newer antibiotics are probably safe for a mother and developing child, there is no way to be sure. This is a catch-22 situation: the antibiotic cannot be tested on pregnant women because it has not been prescribed to them before, and it cannot be prescribed to pregnant women because it has not been tested on them before.

The dosage of all antibiotics should be adjusted for the weight of the patient, but generally only pediatricians, whose patients come in a variety of sizes, pay attention to this detail. Adults commonly—but nevertheless ill-advisedly—get the same dose regardless of their size; whether they are 4 foot 10 inches and weigh 90 pounds, or 6 foot 8 and weigh 300 pounds, they take the same amount of medication. This is not the best way to treat patients, since some may be getting too much medication and others not enough.

The dosage of antibiotics should also be adjusted—that is, reduced—if either the kidneys or the liver is not functioning well. For people with kidney disease, including those on dialysis, the dosage of most antibiotics needs to be adjusted downward according to the amount of remaining function. This is because most antibiotics are excreted from the body by the kidneys, and if this organ system is not working properly, the levels of antibiotics in the blood begin to back up and may exceed the toxicity threshold. Other antibiotics are handled predominantly by the liver; these must be given in reduced dosages if that organ is severely damaged.

In this chapter we've seen how antibiotics work and what the possible side effects of antibiotic therapy are. In the next chapter we'll look more closely at how antibiotic therapy is administered, and we'll consider some of the controversies surrounding the treatment of Lyme disease.

Treating Lyme Disease: What Works and What Doesn't

7

- The pediatrician was right: Julia did feel better by the fourth day of taking doxycycline, and over the next week her rash faded. The pediatrician told Julia's mother to make sure that the child took the antibiotic for the entire three weeks, explaining that it took longer to treat Lyme disease than most other common infections, and she did not want Julia to risk having the disease return later. Julia finished the complete course of therapy and started school again without any trouble in the fall.

- Werner's headache and arm pain decreased after a few days of treatment, but it was several weeks before the strength of the muscles on the right side of his face had substantially improved. Werner eventually graduated with high honors, but because he was afraid of becoming re-infected it was some time before he went hiking in the woods around Vienna again.

- By the time she had taken the full course of oral antibiotics that her physician had initially prescribed, Catherine felt less tired and had fewer muscle aches, but her knee remained swollen and painful. For another month, then, she received additional antibiotic treatment, this time intravenous ceftriaxone once a day, but this treatment had no effect on her knee pain or disability.

  During Catherine's next appointment her rheumatologist wondered aloud whether she was one of those people whose Lyme arthritis does not substantially improve with further antibiotic therapy. He recommended that she undergo two additional laboratory tests to determine whether this was the case. He acknowledged that the tests were expensive and probably were not essential for her care, but the alternative was another course of antibiotics. The rheumatologist was fairly confident that more antibiotics would not be of benefit, and the two additional tests would help to confirm this. Catherine was a person who "liked to get to the bottom of things," and since the tests were unlikely to be more expensive than the intravenous antibiotics, she agreed to have the procedures.

The first test, which was performed at a proficient laboratory in another state, was a PCR assay of fluid obtained from Catherine's swollen knee. The results showed that there was no evidence of *Borrelia burgdorferi* cells remaining in the joint. The second specialized test was performed on some of Catherine's white blood cells. Her physician explained that this test was similar to the test that was performed before a person received an organ or bone marrow transplant, to find a donor with the closest match. The results of the second test showed that Catherine's white blood cells had a feature in common with the cells of other people with this predisposition to a longer-lasting arthritis.

In sum, the results of these two tests indicated that it would be pointless for Catherine to take more antibiotics. She was instead treated with the arthritis drug hydroxychloroquine (Plaquenil) to relieve the pain and to reduce the inflammation. A few weeks later she needed an operation under local anesthesia to remove some of the thickened tissue from her knee. Gradually, over several months, the knee became less painful and swollen, and by the end of the year Catherine was on the golf course again.

■ After returning home and going back to work, Roy did not have any more difficulties with his heart. But he tired more easily during the day, and sometimes his joints and muscles ached. He had trouble concentrating on the technical articles he had to read, often needing to read the same sentence over and over just to understand it. He told the infectious disease specialist on a follow-up visit that he felt as he had when he was getting over hepatitis in the army. "I just don't have as much physical and mental energy as I used to," he said. His physician told Roy that some people experience a prolonged convalescence after Lyme disease and that it was not something to be concerned about. Roy accepted this explanation for about a week but then felt increasingly frustrated about his fatigue and the mental fogginess. He wondered whether something else could be done.

After Roy mentioned this at work, a colleague told him that her sister had this type of Lyme disease, too, and that she had been helped by a physician who had treated her with antibiotics for six months. Roy thought that anything would be better than what he was feeling and made an appointment with the other physician. After examining Roy, the physician told Roy that he was still infected and needed more antibiotics. He started Roy on clarithromycin (Biaxin) and said that he should continue taking it for at least three months. Initially Roy felt a little improved, but by the end of the first month he concluded that he was hundreds of dollars poorer but not any better off. He stopped taking the antibiotics and instead took a long cruise with his family. He felt better when he returned from the trip, but it would be several more weeks before he could at last say he was "100 percent" again.

In the examples I've discussed, the condition of all four people improved—some sooner, some later. Julia, Werner, Catherine, and Roy are not representative of every single person with *B. burgdorferi* infection, but they do illustrate some of the diverse ways in which the infection manifests itself and responds to treatment. We know that, like Julia, most people with Lyme disease are diagnosed at an early stage, such as when the erythema migrans rash emerges, and most of them respond uneventfully to antibiotic treatment. The consternations and controversies about Lyme disease management for the most part aren't concerned with the more straightforward cases like these but are focused on cases like Catherine's and Roy's, in which antibiotics either fail or only partially return the person to health. If there are flurries of dissension regarding the treatment of acute Lyme disease, a tempest of conflict can be said to surround the treatment of chronic disease.

An Overview of Lyme Disease Treatment

As the financial concerns of managed care systems, health maintenance organizations, and governments increasingly determine the direction of medical care, cost disparities between different antibiotic therapies undoubtedly will assume greater importance in treatment decisions. But for the present, cost, while not disregarded, in most cases takes a back seat to two other considerations: which treatment is most effective, and which treatment is least harmful? If they know that an insurance plan will cover all or most of the tab for office visits and treatments, patients seldom ask how much the treatment will cost. By contrast, people without health insurance or other financial means often consider cost to be the critical factor in choosing a treatment for Lyme disease.

In treating most people with *B. burgdorferi* infection, the physician, or the physician in collaboration with the patient, is free to pick among the several choices. Some physicians have treated Lyme disease by prescribing a few days of an oral tetracycline or penicillin; others have treated the disease with several months' worth of intravenous antibiotic followed by continuous oral antibiotics.

In the future, case managers of insurance plans, other third party payers, and health maintenance organizations may demand a more assiduous accounting of the costs and benefits of the various Lyme disease therapies. How much better, they may ask, is a course of intravenous antibiotics costing seven thousand dollars than treatment with an oral generic antibiotic that costs less than a dollar for each dose? The physician's response conceivably could be that using the intravenous antibiotic raises the cure rate from 90 to 95 percent, or from 95 to 99 percent, or from 99 to 100 percent. But right now, the physician and the experts that he or she might call on to corroborate this view cannot be that precise. And indeed, for many forms of Lyme disease, more expensive intravenous therapy may offer no advantage for the patient.

While the amount of useful information about Lyme disease treatment has increased, much of the therapy prescribed for this condition remains empirical, and our knowledge of the results of therapy remains anecdotal—that is, individual reports of relief obtained after taking a particular medicine. Overall, more is known about the harm antibiotics can cause than is known about the effectiveness of different treatment plans. There is little debate on what constitutes harm— diarrhea, hives, a falling white blood cell count, and gall bladder blockage are not subtle symptoms—but measuring the "effectiveness" of a Lyme disease therapy is another matter.

The least ambiguous way to assess therapeutic success is to determine whether the microorganism—be it virus, bacterium, fungus, or parasite—has been eliminated from the treated patient: the patient's lungs contained the tuberculosis bacterium before treatment and not afterwards; the agent of dysentery was identified in a sample of feces before treatment but not afterwards.

Medical investigators have cultured skin samples from people before and after antibiotic treatment of erythema migrans and have shown that therapy has eliminated the spirochetes from that site. But, as we saw in Chapter 5, this degree of microbiologic precision cannot be achieved at present in most cases of chronic Lyme disease. Researchers who are studying the success of antibiotic treatment under these circumstances are relatively dependent on more subjective evidence: the person's symptoms and sense of well-being. Without a doubt, the evaluation of how the person *feels* is what ultimately counts most, but researchers are usually more comfortable with statistics from the microbiology laboratory than they are with patients' self-reports.

Keeping this set of cautions in mind, we can begin to explore the different ways that *B. burgdorferi* infection is treated. While acknowledging that exceptions are inevitable, we can describe treatment in general terms this way:

- Oral antibiotics are used in the treatment of early localized infection, early disseminated infection, and late infection (i.e., chronic Lyme disease) when there is no evidence of invasion of the nervous system. The oral antibiotics most commonly recommended for early disease are amoxicillin and doxycycline. Other oral drugs used are cefuroxime, cefixime, azithromycin, clarithromycin, and minocycline.
- Intravenous antibiotics are reserved for use in the treatment of early disseminated infection, or late infection in which the heart, eye, or nervous system is affected. They are also used when an adequate trial of an oral antibiotic has failed. The most commonly recommended intravenous antibiotics are cefotaxime, ceftriaxone, and penicillin.

Two of the "gray areas" in the decision matrix are arthritis and Bell's palsy (nerve weakness on one or both sides of the face). Some physicians would treat these conditions from the beginning with intravenous drugs, while others would try oral treatment first. Many of those who treat early disseminated and chronic disease initially with oral antibiotics do so only after performing a spinal tap to see if there is evidence of brain involvement. If there are increased white blood cells or protein in the cerebrospinal fluid, then intravenous antibiotics are used.

Choosing between Intravenous and Oral Antibiotics
Advantages of Intravenous Antibiotics

Setting cost and convenience aside for the moment, what reasons are there for using an intravenous instead of an oral antibiotic? First, the most appropriate antibiotic may not be suitable for oral use. In order to work, some drugs have to bypass the stomach, and this is most easily accomplished by directly administering the drug into a vein through an intravenous needle ("i.v.") or into a muscle through a "shot." If given orally, such an antibiotic may be broken down by the acid or other substances in the stomach, or it may not be sufficiently absorbed into the blood from the intestine. Some antibiotics cannot be given orally because when given by that route they cause unacceptable nausea, diarrhea, or other noxious effects. (Conversely, some antibiotics are restricted to oral administration because they are too irritating to be given by i.v. or injection. The intestinal tract can tolerate more than the nerve endings in our blood vessels and muscles can.)

For any antibiotic that is effective and well tolerated, regardless of which route it is given by, the second reason for choosing vein over mouth is the higher concentration of the drug that can usually be achieved by intravenous route. Similarly high levels might be achieved if large enough amounts were given by mouth, but achieving this concentration by the oral route often creates intolerable or even dangerous side effects. What's critical here is not so much the level or concentration of antibiotic in the blood, since all of the antibiotics routinely used for oral treatment achieve sufficiently high levels in the blood to kill or inhibit *B. burgdorferi*. (These blood levels are usually adequate to inhibit spirochetes in the skin and some other tissues, too.) Rather, in certain cases the amount of antibiotic in the brain and in the CSF, the fluid around it, becomes critical.

For an antibiotic to work on spirochetes in the brain, the concentration in the blood has to be roughly ten times as great as the level desired for the brain. For example, if *B. burgdorferi* is inhibited by one microgram (a thirty-thousandth of an ounce) of an antibiotic dissolved in a milliliter (about a thousandth of a quart), the blood concentration of the antibiotic should be at least ten micrograms per milliliter to assure inhibitory levels of antibiotic in brain or cerebrospinal fluid. Penicillin by mouth in tolerated doses might reach two or three micrograms per milliliter of blood, but this level is not high enough to have the desired effect in the brain.

A more speculative and, as yet, less compelling rationale for intravenous therapy is the concern that some spirochetes are less accessible to antibiotics by virtue of the bacteria's tendency to locate itself within cells or use other evasive tactics. The reasoning is that higher levels of antibiotic, attainable only by the i.v. route, are required to snuff out these elusive remnants of infection. Only a small proportion of the blood's antibiotic may reach the spirochetes in their hideouts, and consequently, the levels in the blood must be higher to begin with. As discussed in the preceding chapter, some antibiotics are particularly good at getting into cells, but these antibiotics tend to be ones that are used orally. For the routinely used intravenous antibiotics, such as ceftriaxone, there usually is a substantial gradient between what is outside and what is inside the cells.

Given the acknowledged limitations of oral antibiotics in providing for adequate levels in the brain, the usual strategy has been to treat documented or suspected brain involvement in Lyme disease with intravenous antibiotics. This policy is not unique to Lyme disease. Intravenous or intramuscular antibiotics have for years been recommended for most infections of the brain. People with meningitis (infection of the covering of the brain) or with abscesses of the brain are routinely treated with intravenous antibiotics in the hospital.

Today's standard of practice does not rule out a day when brain infections will be more routinely treated by oral antibiotics. The expense and inconvenience of giving intravenous drugs provides motivation for the development of more effective orally delivered therapies. This may even be possible now, with currently available antibiotics, but not much work has been done with this approach. The doses would have to be high enough to yield satisfactory brain levels but not so high that people cannot stand the side effects. Experience tells us that it is difficult to achieve this balance, but to make the attempt may be appropriate in selected situations—as has been demonstrated by some investigators who used doxycycline at twice the usual dose to successfully treat brain involvement by *B. burgdorferi*.

Another way that higher brain levels of antibiotics can be achieved is to combine one of the orally administered penicillins, such as amoxicillin, with another drug, probenecid (Benemid), that boosts the antibiotic's levels in various tissues and fluids. When probenecid is used with a penicillin, the antibiotic level in the blood is about twice what it is without the adjunct medicine. Whether this boost is enough to warrant the addition of another medication, with its own attendant risks, remains to be tested in a clinical trial.

One advantage of intravenous antibiotics is that they are usually given by a nurse who, by nature, training, and selection, is punctual. Missing a dose is seldom a problem for inpatients, and in the hospital setting it doesn't make a great deal of difference whether an antibiotic is given two or three times a day—or four to eight. Less frequent dosing means lower daily costs for needles, tubing, bottles, and labor, but this savings is often offset by the higher per-unit costs of newer antibiotics, such as ceftriaxone and cefotaxime (which cost more because they are under patent protection).

Other Factors in the Choice between Oral and Intravenous Antibiotics

By contrast, treatment by mouth is simple: a pill once, twice, at most four times a day. And oral antibiotics are one of the cheaper kinds of medical treatment. Doxycycline and amoxicillin, the commonly prescribed oral treatments for early Lyme disease, are available in generic forms. These antibiotics cost less than a dollar for a full day's dose. (Antibiotics such as cefuroxime and azithromycin, which are still under patent protection and consequently are not available in generic versions, cost several times as much.) But there are also disadvantages to administering antibiotics by mouth.

Oral antibiotics are usually self-administered by people who have not been admitted to the hospital, and a common reason for the drugs' failure to work is the patient's or family's forgetfulness. Remembering to take a pill three or four times a day for several days to weeks is difficult, even for compulsive people. Studies have shown that about 40 percent of people are not able to comply with a four-times-a-day dosing schedule. Less frequent dosing means less chance of missing a dose, and taking a pill once or twice a day is easily incorporated into a routine of swallowing vitamin pills or brushing one's teeth. Those marketing many of the new oral antibiotics introduced in recent years boast that their products require less frequent dosing than, say, penicillin or tetracycline. Two of the most recently marketed antibiotics are taken but once a day.

Besides patient noncompliance, another disadvantage of oral antibiotics is their longer journey from medicine bottle to site of infection. Intravenous drugs, in contrast, run from the bottle directly into the blood. The gastrointestinal component of the effectiveness of orally administered antibiotics has already been described, and explains why drug designers work to maximize absorption of an antibiotic from the gastrointestinal tract. The absorption of many early antibiotics, including plain penicillin and tetracycline, was determined in large measure by the contents of the intestinal tract. For example, tetracycline's ability to move from stomach to blood is affected by the presence of food to such an extent that this antibiotic should not be taken within an hour or two of a meal. Tetracycline should also not be consumed at the same time as antacids or milk. The aluminum in some antacids and the calcium in milk binds to tetracycline and effectively inactivates it. One reason that physicians prefer amoxicillin over penicillin for oral treatment is that amoxicillin is absorbed more efficiently from the gastrointestinal tract.

Then there's the lesser convenience of i.v. therapy, and more important, the danger of a superimposed infection associated with it. The process and paraphernalia required for administering an antibiotic by vein make it more complicated than administering an oral drug. For intravenous therapy, a needle or plastic catheter must first be placed in a vein in the arm or some other location. Most people, because of inexperience or squeamishness, could not do this themselves, and so a second person trained and skilled in this procedure is needed. Next, a length of plastic tubing is connected to the inserted needle or catheter. Finally, the antibiotic powder is dissolved in a sterile liquid and the antibiotic is dripped in, along with dilute salt or sugar water, through the tubing. All these steps are performed under sterile conditions. A specialized pump controls the infusion of the antibiotic into the patient. To prevent toxic levels of the antibiotic in the blood, care has to be taken that the antibiotic does not run in too quickly.

The inserted needle or catheter, which is usually left in place between treatments, provides an opening that can allow bacteria and fungi to enter the body. Some patients have longer-lasting tubes placed deep into a shoulder or chest vein by a small operation. A superimposed infection of the vein and blood is a serious possible complication of intravenous therapy. A number of different microorganisms may infect the i.v. site, some of them resistant to multiple antibiotics and therefore difficult to treat. Some people receiving intravenous therapy for Lyme disease have suffered life-threatening secondary infections.

Outpatient Intravenous Therapy

A person who is undergoing i.v. therapy outside the hospital is fairly free to pursue a normal lifestyle. Once or twice a day the person must sit or lie down during the drug's delivery, but thereafter he or she can resume daily activities. Sometimes patients or family members learn to administer the antibiotic or other medicine themselves. Until about ten years ago, however, this was seldom a possibility. A hospitalized person, or inpatient, often had to remain in the hospital for several weeks just to receive an antibiotic administered by vein. Now the option exists of receiving intravenous treatments as an outpatient at the hospital or clinic, or at home.

Several factors have brought about what has been an exponential growth in this area of medicine. Two were technological. The fact that newer intravenous antibiotics require less frequent dosing than, say, penicillin, made therapy outside the hospital more convenient and therefore more feasible. And the development of small, portable pumps made it possible to control the flow of the intravenous fluids.

For some time there has been the expectation that home- or clinic-based therapy would be less expensive than hospital-based therapy. Although this will likely come to be so in the future, and this expectation remains a major force in the direction of more outpatient treatments, at this time the final charges to the patient, and ultimately to the third-party payer, for intravenous antibiotic therapy are often about the same whether the patient is hospitalized or at home. One week's worth of intravenous therapy as an outpatient costs between two thousand and four thousand dollars.

The excessively high cost for this care is in part due to a lack of regulation in this exploding field of medicine. Only a minority of states license companies that provide home intravenous care, and these companies have been known to mark up prices for medicines and materials unreasonably. Some have forced families to pay for leftover but untouched medicines after the patient has died. In other situations physicians have received "consultation fees," which are essentially kickbacks, for referring patients to companies providing home i.v. care. And some physicians have held a financial interest in the home i.v. therapy companies to which they refer patients; this qualifies as a conflict of interest on the physician's part. These abuses are beginning to decline as states begin to regulate the activities of the companies and the prescribing physicians. Insurance companies and other third-party payers have also become more alert to overcharges and other dubious maneuvers that are used to increase profit margins.

The many attractive features of home-based i.v. therapy notwithstanding, most patients who receive intravenous antibiotic therapy for one infection or another still do so in a hospital. They may need hospitalization for as long as treatment continues because they are too sick to leave. Some people are well enough to manage at home without full-time nursing help, but the logistics of outpatient i.v.

therapy make it impractical, too costly, or unsafe for them. Home i.v. therapy is not recommended if

- neither the patient nor other household members, if there are any, is physically or mentally capable of caring for the needle or catheter that is left in the patient between treatments;
- the antibiotic has to be given so often during the day that the home setting provides little advantage over a hospital setting;
- the community care facility or the medically indigent care facility lacks the resources and wherewithal to provide outpatient i.v. therapy; or
- the patient is an intravenous user of illicit drugs such as cocaine or heroin.

For most people with Lyme disease, however, home-based therapy is practical, and they are good candidates for it. For one thing, most people with Lyme disease, even at its worst, are not so sick that hospitalization is required. And tests for evaluation and diagnosis can be done on an outpatient basis. Patients such as Roy, who was monitored in the cardiac care unit, and Werner, who initially had an extensive neurologic workup in the hospital, are the exception.

A second reason that people with Lyme disease so often can be treated with i.v. antibiotics as outpatients is the demographics of the group most at risk for the disease: they tend to be middle- to upper-income individuals who live with other family members, are comparatively well educated, and are motivated to participate actively in their own care. Moreover, most cases of Lyme disease occur in the densely populated Northeast and upper Midwest. Even if the patient lives in the countryside, a suburban or urban area is close at hand, where there are numerous facilities for home and outpatient clinic treatments.

Although numbers are hard to come by, it seems that outpatient therapy for Lyme disease provides much business for home i.v. care companies in some areas of the country. Others who benefit financially are the makers of the commonly used antibiotics, especially Hoffman–La Roche's ceftriaxone, which with its once-daily dosage is the drug of first choice for home therapy. Even for conventional treatments, patients receive two to four weeks of intravenous therapy at a cost of thousands of dollars.

Some home i.v. care companies have such a strong interest in Lyme disease that they have helped sponsor newsletters for patient support groups, some of which advocate longer-than-conventional treatments for chronic Lyme disease. Even less ethically defensible is the practice of some home i.v. companies or their representatives that provide telephone "hot lines" on Lyme disease. Persons calling these hot lines are sometimes referred to physicians who prescribe extended intravenous therapies.

Lining up against long treatments are those who ultimately pay for much of it: insurance companies, governmental institutions, and health management organizations (HMOs). Increasingly, these companies and other third-party payers, as they have seen their expenses for Lyme disease treatment escalate, refuse to cover more than one month of intravenous treatment for Lyme disease. They and their medical consultants argue that treatment beyond this limit is seldom necessary and that for most routine cases it is experimental and of no proven benefit.

Many people treated for months with home i.v. therapy face huge bills, sometimes more than one hundred thousand dollars. Desperate and vulnerable in their search for relief of their symptoms, some people are willing to pay amounts like this. Others, frustrated or angry at what they perceive to be a lack of appreciation of the nature of their disease, have brought suit against the insurance companies for full reimbursement of extended intravenous antibiotic treatments. Some individuals and patient advocacy groups have petitioned and lobbied their state legislatures to force the companies to pay for long-term antibiotic therapy.

To make better sense of a medical controversy that inspires litigation and political activism, we need first to explore other aspects of therapy with antibiotics.

If Enough Is Good, Is More Better?

Once an antibiotic in the blood, tissue, or CSF reaches a level that kills or inhibits the spirochetes that cause Lyme disease, even much higher concentrations of the antibiotics do not speed up the spiro-chetes' death. (Some antibiotics do have this additive effect, but they are not used to treat Lyme disease.) Therefore, there is no advantage to giving larger doses than is necessary. More side effects would be the only consequence. But the timing of the doses is important in making therapy as effective as possible. The antibiotic may reach the critical level, but if it does not remain above that level for a certain amount of time during the day, the antibiotic may fail. This is be-cause, although the bacteria may be temporarily slowed in growing, and some of them may even be killed, they will regain ground or even gain additional ground once the antibiotic level falls below the threshold for inhibition.

If the antibiotic is dripped in slowly and continuously through a vein, the level is certain to be kept high enough for a long enough period. An alternative has been to give the antibiotic orally but fre-quently, in the range of four to eight times a day. For periodic treat-ment the dose is large enough that the antibiotic level in the body seldom if ever drops below the minimal effective concentration. If it drops below the threshold level, it does not do so for so long that the bacteria begin growing again. Knocked out by an antibiotic, a bac-terium takes an hour or more to recover.

An extreme variation of the periodic treatment approach is what has been called "pulse" therapy, in which antibiotic is given as usual for several days running and then stopped for a period of time, usu-ally one day or a few days. The rationale given for pulse therapy is that partial recovery of the bacteria is in fact desirable. The propo-nents point out the successful use of pulse dosing in the treatment of cancer. Because growing cells, be they cancer cells or bacteria, are most susceptible to chemotherapy, it makes sense, according to this theory, to allow the bacteria to begin growing again. At the point this begins to happen, the next pulse of antibiotic might kill larger numbers of them. Compelling as this argument is, there have been few studies of the effectiveness of this type of treatment for any type of infection. The effectiveness of pulse therapy at this point remains unproven for Lyme disease.

Penicillin is an example of an antibiotic that must be given either continuously or at frequent intervals. Newer antibiotics do not necessarily surpass penicillin in their abilities to kill *B. burgdorferi*, but some of them have a practical advantage over penicillin and other older antibiotics in that they need to be administered less often during the day—as infrequently as once a day in the case of ceftriaxone and azithromycin. This attractive feature is due to their greater "staying power" in the body. In comparison to penicillin and tetracycline, these long-lasting antibiotics are not as quickly eliminated through the urine or metabolized in the blood or the organs.

Are Two Antibiotics Better than One?

If uncommonly high doses of a single antibiotic provide no noticeable benefit but do cause uncomfortable side effects, one option is to treat persistent infections with conventional doses of two antibiotics in combination. The individual antibiotics in the combination can be additive or even synergistic (meaning that the effect of the two drugs together is greater than would be predicted from how they perform when administered alone). For example, assume that antibiotic A kills a bacterium at a minimum concentration of ten micrograms per milliliter and that antibiotic B kills it at a concentration of one hundred micrograms. If the combination of antibiotics A and B killed the bacteria in concentrations of two and twenty, respectively, this would be an example of a synergistic combination. The use of antibiotics A and B together would provide effective treatment with lower doses of each of the drugs, thus possibly avoiding some unpleasant side effects of higher doses.

Although combinations are used with good effect for other infections, notably some serious infections of the heart valves and the lungs, little is known about how useful this approach is for Lyme disease. A drug widely sold as a combination of two antibiotics, trimethoprim-sulfamethoxazole, is effective in treating a variety of mild to serious infections but is not at all effective for *B. burgdorferi* infections. A drug combination conceivably could be of benefit in difficult Lyme disease cases, but there is no laboratory evidence to support this approach at this time. Empirical combination therapy can also backfire, because an undesirable consequence of using two antibiotics is that one of them sometimes blocks the effect of the other. Physicians traditionally have avoided combinations of a tetracycline with a penicillin because the tetracycline may interfere with the killing action of the penicillin.

Another justification for using more than one antibiotic at a time is to prevent the emergence of antibiotic-resistant bacteria during treatment. This strategy is routinely used in treating people who have tuberculosis. Someone with an active case of tuberculosis may have huge numbers of bacteria in the lungs. Chances are that at least one member of the bacterial population is already resistant to an antibiotic. If only one antibiotic is used, the unresistant bacteria will die, but that one resistant mutant bacterium will grow to two, four, eight, and so on until it has replaced the antibiotic-susceptible cells. The patient is just as sick but now has a bacterial population that cannot be wiped out with an antibiotic. When two or more antibiotics are used in combination, however, one of the antibiotics will kill a mutant that is resistant to the other—if the two antibiotics work in different ways. The odds that a single bacterium would become resistant to two or more different antibiotics at the same time are very low.

Is this experience with tuberculosis relevant to Lyme disease, especially its more troublesome chronic form, which is suspected by some of being resistant to antibiotics? Probably not. Mutants of *B. burgdorferi* that are resistant to standard therapies have not been detected in the environment or in patients. Different strains of these bacteria from various locales in the world vary up to tenfold in their susceptibilities to some antibiotics in the laboratory, but this amount of variation is not worrisome. Truly resistant bacteria usually differ from their susceptible counterparts by a hundred- or thousandfold.

A more instructive analogy than tuberculosis may be syphilis, another serious spirochete infection of humans. Like Lyme disease, syphilis in its chronic phase does not typically feature large numbers of microorganisms in the body. Relatively few spirochetes spark damage in both types of infection. When bacterial populations are small like this, the chance that resistant mutants are already present in an infected person before treatment starts is low. If it takes the presence of at least one hundred million bacteria for there to be an expectation of finding one or more resistant mutants, then antibiotic resistance is unlikely if there are only a total of ten million spirochetes in a person. And because all of the infecting bacteria in a person are probably susceptible to the antibiotic to begin with, we would not expect that one or more of the bacteria would upon exposure to the antibiotic suddenly change their genes to become resistant. As Charles Darwin and many others have said, that is not how evolution works.

Syphilis has been successfully treated for half a century with penicillin administered on its own. Penicillin-resistant mutants have not been noted in the millions of people who have been treated for syphilis with this antibiotic. And if, as we suspect, the treatment history of syphilis is a useful guide, then taking two or three antibiotics at a time for the treatment of Lyme disease is unnecessary.

Is Longer Better than Shorter?

Few practitioners argue about the size of the doses of antibiotics given to treat Lyme disease in its different stages. More controversial is the appropriate *duration* of therapy, especially for chronic Lyme disease. There are natural limits on treatment decisions about doses: below a certain level an antibiotic will not work, and above a certain concentration side effects increase. Too little antibiotic, the person remains infected; too much antibiotic, the person becomes sick in another way. The possibilities for treatment duration, however, are literally endless, ranging from one dose to lifelong consumption. A single dose of an antibiotic cures some bacterial infections, such as gonorrhea or an uncomplicated urinary tract infection. Other diseases, such as tuberculosis, require months to years of treatment for a cure. Some people with leprosy or some deep-seated, inoperable infections take antibiotics for the rest of their lives; their infection can be controlled but never eradicated.

Is Lyme disease closer to the gonorrhea model or to the leprosy model in terms of the length of therapy required for cure? Of these two infections, gonorrhea is closer, but "strep" throat may be a better analogy to early Lyme disease. Streptococcus infection of the throat and tonsils is effectively treated with a week to two of antibiotics—

more than a day but less than a lifetime. If streptococci remain in the throat, there is a chance of relapse and of more serious sequelae, such as rheumatic fever or kidney disease. And if any *B. burgdorferi* survive antibiotic therapy for early Lyme disease, chronic Lyme disease could develop in the future.

Experiments in the laboratory provide reasons to be confident that treatment for early Lyme disease should last for days or a few weeks rather than months. Several studies have now shown that even a few days of various antibiotics given to mice, hamsters, and gerbils are sufficient to eliminate all evidence of infection with *B. burgdorferi*. The laboratory animals were infected, and once the infection was established they were treated for different periods of time with an antibiotic. After the antibiotic treatment was completed and a suitable time was allowed to pass so that any remaining antibiotic would "wash out," the animals were humanely put to sleep and their blood and different tissues were cultured or subjected to PCR analysis. By these methods even a handful of spirochetes remaining after the antibiotics should have been detectable in the animals. But at the end of the experiment the animals receiving antibiotic doses comparable to what a human would get were found to be free of infection.

Treatment of Early Disease

Valuable as these laboratory experiments are, the most meaningful information comes from studying people with the disease. A picture (albeit still fuzzy in many areas) is emerging as a result of the increasing number of clinical trials on the treatment of early Lyme disease. The picture is sharpened a bit by the cumulative experiences of thousands of physicians in North America, Europe, Russia, and Asia who have by now treated people with *B. burgdorferi* infections. These trials and experiences have essentially confirmed the first report of some Swedish physicians of more than forty years ago: antibiotics are effective treatment for erythema migrans and other manifestations of early Lyme disease. To be specific, about nineteen out of every twenty people treated with certain antibiotics for acute *B. burgdorferi* infection benefit from the treatment. Their rashes fade sooner with antibiotics than without. The spirochetes disappear from the skin where erythema migrans occurred. People begin to feel better earlier when they are treated than when they are not. There is a significantly lower risk of late arthritis or neurologic disease if early disease is treated with antibiotics rather than just observed by the physician.

The antibiotics demonstrated to be effective for treatment of early disease are penicillin, tetracycline, doxycycline, amoxicillin, penicillin, erythromycin, cefuroxime, and azithromycin. Penicillin and tetracycline, the two earliest antibiotics used for erythema migrans, have largely been replaced by amoxicillin and doxycycline, respectively, because these drugs are absorbed better by the intestinal tract and require less frequent dosing. Erythromycin was less effective than penicillin or tetracycline, and now it is generally used only in young children, pregnant or nursing women, and those who are allergic to penicillins. Tetracyclines and some of the newer, less thoroughly tested antibiotics are not administered to young children (because they stain the developing permanent teeth) or to pregnant or nursing women.

The duration of most treatments has ranged from ten days to three weeks. Going from ten to twenty-one days of therapy may increase the cure rate to more than 95 percent. (Because of expected differences in patients' compliance, it is difficult to achieve a 100-percent success rate with self-administered oral antibiotics for any infection.) But let's consider: If three weeks of therapy is better than a week and a half, perhaps four weeks of therapy is better than three. If four weeks is better than three, then perhaps five or six weeks ought to be the gold standard. And since the complications of chronic encephalopathy or arthritis can drastically change a person's life, shouldn't people minimize their chances of getting chronic Lyme disease?

In fact, the principal goal of treatment of early disease is this exactly: to stop the progression of the infection to a chronic disease. Relief of symptoms is important, of course, but the truth is that erythema migrans and other manifestations of acute *B. burgdorferi* infection usually resolve themselves without antibiotics. Even so, extending therapy beyond a certain duration will not bring added benefit.

Needlessly prolonging treatment only runs up expenses and increases the risk of side effects or a drug allergy.

That having been said, it's important to note that there are some
situations in which early Lyme disease may be treated more aggres-
sively, either with four weeks instead of two to three weeks of oral
therapy or with an intravenous antibiotic. When the physician suspects that infection has spread from the skin to other parts of the
body, such as the brain, the heart, or the joints, then longer treatment
may be used. The symptoms, signs, and laboratory evidence of brain
involvement (described in Chapter 1) without question call for intravenous therapy, as in Werner's case. If the heart is affected, someone
like Roy will probably be hospitalized and treated as an inpatient
with i.v. antibiotics. Other indications of widespread early disease are
arthritis affecting several joints, multiple erythema migrans lesions
on the skin, painful, burning sensations of one or more limbs, and
the combination of fever and severe fatigue.

The success rate for oral antibiotics appears to be somewhat lower
in people with early disseminated infection than in people with a localized acute infection, that is, a single erythema migrans rash, but
we have less information about therapeutic effectiveness in these situations, since fewer people with early disseminated disease have been
included in the clinical trials to date. What information is available
suggests that people with evidence of dissemination at the time treatment starts are more apt to require another course of antibiotics or to
endure late disease. The risk of chronic infection for these people is less
than for people whose acute infection has not been treated, however.

The people who take longest to fully recover from specific organ
involvement in early disseminated disease are those whose nerves
have been badly damaged. This is because it can take months for the
long lengths of nerve fibers to be replaced by new growth. Some
people do not ever recover function completely. This can be particularly tragic when the nerve weakness is located in the face.

The Post–Lyme Disease Syndrome

Some people with early Lyme disease, whether it is localized or
disseminated, suffer in a more generalized, less organ-specific way

long after antibiotic therapy has been completed. The rash may be just a memory, the heart is beating regularly again, the joints are once again limber enough for tennis, but everything is still not right. Roy is an example of someone with a prolonged convalescence.

As many as one-quarter to one-third of the people with early disease continue to suffer some symptoms and debility after antibiotics have been completed. Their overall health is better, but they may continue to lack energy, become easily fatigued, and have recurrent muscle and joint aches and headaches that last for a few weeks to several months. Some complain of mental sluggishness and difficulty in concentrating. Like Roy, they do not begin to feel "100 percent" as soon as they had hoped they would. If this condition lasts long enough, it may also be called chronic fatigue syndrome or fibromyalgia. (These disorders are considered in Chapter 8.)

A post-infection syndrome is a characteristic collection of symptoms following a documented or suspected infection. This phenomenon is not unique to Lyme disease. People experience similar debilitating symptoms as an aftermath of many types of infection, including influenza, hepatitis, and infectious mononucleosis. In most of these instances the infectious agent is either eliminated or no longer multiplying. The syndrome may be due to a prolonged activation of the immune system by the bacterium or virus—the infection may be turned off, but the immune system is still turned on. Cytokines and nervous system chemicals that increase in numbers and amounts during infection may have enduring effects. When some cytokines are used as drugs themselves and given to people as treatments for cancer and other conditions, the patients experience fatigue, muscle aches, and difficulties in concentrating. Such symptoms are similar to those of treated Lyme disease.

The personality or preinfection mood of the infected person may also have a bearing on the time required for convalescence. The effect of a person's mental state on infection outcome was studied in two situations. One was a college in which students had taken a personality test at the start of the year. Then those who came down with infectious mononucleosis were examined and further questioned. In the second study an epidemic of influenza was tracked in a group of people who had taken psychological tests just before the epidemic hit. In both studies it was found that people with a predisposition toward depression and those who had a less optimistic outlook took longer to convalesce from infection than those without these traits.

Whatever the post-infection syndrome is called, and regardless of what effect mood or cytokines may have on its evolution and duration, the practical issue in an individual case is whether these lingering symptoms represent continued infection by B. burgdorferi or the person's response to an infection that has effectively been halted. If it is suspected that an infection is still active, another course of antibiotics is needed. But if the bacteria have already been inhibited or killed, additional antibiotics would not be expected to be of benefit, except through their placebo or nonspecific effects.

The accumulated experience with other infections suggests that a delayed resolution of the body's activated state (and not a residual active infection) is the basis for the post-infection syndromes. In the Lyme disease experience, some patients with persistent generalized symptoms that cannot be associated with a specific place, such as a knee joint, do benefit from another round of antibiotics. But most do not. The few who do appear to improve with additional antibiotics may have been inadequately treated the first time around—for instance, with less than two weeks of antibiotics for localized disease or less than three weeks for disseminated disease.

Without evidence one way or another, it's impossible to say conclusively whether people whose symptoms persist following treatment are at higher risk of Lyme disease reactivation than are those with faster recoveries. There are conflicting reports about the long-term outcomes of people who have been treated for early Lyme disease. Some investigators report that roughly one-third of former patients continue, even years later, to have joint complaints or subtle difficulties in their memory function and ability to concentrate. Others have found persistent or recurrent problems more than a year after initial treatment to be rare among appropriately treated people.

Post–Lyme Disease Syndrome versus Chronic Lyme Disease

Post–Lyme disease syndrome may be confused with chronic Lyme disease, the late form of infection with B. *burgdorferi*. The difference between the two disorders is that most patients with late infection still respond, at least partially, to antibiotic therapy, while patients with the post-infection syndrome usually do not. The distinction may be subtle, though, because patients with true late infection may have received antibiotics in the past, usually in inadequate dosages or durations. In the next section, I deal both with the diagnosis of chronic Lyme disease, which may not be correct, and with cases in which the certainty of persistent infection with B. *burgdorferi* is high. I attempt to discriminate between these situations. We also have to distinguish a case, like Catherine's, in which the micro-organism was likely eliminated by treatment but the arthritis continued. This sounds like post–Lyme disease syndrome, in terms of its lack of response to additional antibiotics, but is still usually considered a manifestation of chronic Lyme disease. Admittedly, this confusion of terms and inexactness of definitions is frustrating, even maddening. Lay persons, health care providers, and scientists alike feel this. Chapter 8 shows that the situation is even more complicated.

Treatment of Chronic Lyme Disease

People who have been told that they have chronic Lyme disease face a difficult choice. They and their families are disconcerted and may be confused by the controversy about how to treat this condition. The controversy is so spirited that physicians who endorse a specific method of treatment have even had their offices picketed, and they have been heckled when they make public presentations. The people doing the picketing and the heckling hold a different view of how Lyme disease should be diagnosed and treated. So many complaints were made about what was perceived to be unfair representation in a government-sponsored scientific conference that previously rejected papers were included at the last moment. This contentiousness over treatment, frustrating for patient and physician alike, is not surprising given the different interpretations of what Lyme disease is and the dispute over the diagnostic process.

The disagreement can be summarized and simplified as follows: Many physicians, mostly based at academic and governmental institutions, have stated in writing and in professional and public presentations that antibiotic treatment of chronic Lyme disease seldom needs to continue for longer than a month. These recommendations are made in current textbooks and in many medical periodicals, as well, and at least one public education group, the American Lyme Disease Foundation, also backs them. (Many physicians in private practice seem to quietly agree with this viewpoint, too, although it is admittedly difficult to monitor this without a formal poll or survey.)

On the other side of the disagreement are several practitioners and some members of patient advocacy groups who believe that treating chronic Lyme disease for longer than a month is justified in many more instances than these textbook recommendations would allow for. At the crux of the disagreement lie different definitions of chronic Lyme disease and different assumptions about what antibiotics can do to *B. burgdorferi* in the body. The differences in definitions of chronic Lyme disease are discussed elsewhere (Chapter 8). The different beliefs about the effects of antibiotics are considered here.

Notwithstanding the intensity of the debate, there are some points of agreement between the two groups. Undeniably, antibiotic treatment shortens the course of many cases of late infection involving the joints and nervous system. This has been shown in controlled medical trials. The human subjects of the study all met strict definitions of Lyme disease and had laboratory test evidence of *B. burgdorferi* infection. People with less compatible symptoms and signs or without antibody evidence of infection were not included in these trials. In the studies, people who received antibiotics intravenously for two to three weeks for their chronic arthritis or neurologic disorder improved in their symptoms and were able to function sooner than those who did not. Approximately half of the people with arthritis and two-thirds of those with neurologic disease were either cured or substantially improved by antibiotic therapy. Again, we can say that people with chronic Lyme disease are better off treated than not treated with antibiotics.

Physicians caring for many Lyme disease patients have noted that even a month of treatment is not curative for a few people with indisputable Lyme disease. This failure could be caused by several things. First, if oral antibiotics are used, the person may miss enough doses so that he or she receives insufficiently high levels of antibiotics for a period of time. Or a few spirochetes may survive a standard course of intravenous therapy because they were not growing—and thus were not susceptible—during the antibiotic period. Some researchers and physicians have suggested that if spirochetes survive within cells during the time of treatment, they might grow again when the antibiotic stops. The penicillin-type antibiotics, though they are excellent at killing *B. burgdorferi*, can do this effectively only if the bacteria are growing and are located outside of cells.

One of the problems in determining whether the spirochetes are still present and alive in such situations, though, is that it is hard to find the microorganisms or traces of microorganisms in people with late disease even *before* treatment, let alone after treatment. The antibody test, usually an ELISA, may be helpful here. If high antibody levels to *B. burgdorferi* are indirect evidence of the spirochete's presence for the original diagnosis, then a declining amount of antibody in the blood can be evidence of a resolution of infection. Once an invading microorganism has been eliminated or controlled, the immune system backs off, and the amount of antibody to the microorganism decreases, as do the numbers of white blood cells that react specifically to the microorganism. This happens in chronic Lyme disease, too, but it can be months to years before there is an unambiguous decline in the amount of antibody in the blood. A definite decrease in the ELISA titer or value from its peak provides reassurance that the infection is no longer active, but the converse is not necessarily true. That is, an unchanging ELISA titer does not mean that the infection continues.

The newly developed PCR assay offers the chance to obtain direct evidence of spirochete tenacity after treatment of chronic Lyme arthritis. Only rarely has *B. burgdorferi* been cultivated from an arthritic joint, but the spirochete's DNA can commonly be detected in the joint fluid or tissue. If after treatment a person has unrelieved joint pain and swelling, then the finding of *B. burgdorferi* DNA in the joint fluids or tissue by PCR indicates that such a person will likely respond wholly or partially to further antibiotic therapy. However, those people who don't have a PCR finding of continuing infection do not benefit from further antibiotic treatment. (The PCR assay remains an experimental assay for Lyme disease, and only a few laboratories in the world are qualified to perform it for this purpose.)

Other people with Lyme arthritis do not perceptibly improve with antibiotics, even after two or more courses, because one form of chronic Lyme arthritis can continue even without living spirochetes. This was Catherine's situation. Her arthritis was unchecked even after two consecutive month-long courses of antibiotics, one of which was given intravenously. The treatment probably helped stop the disease by killing the remaining bacteria. But the autoimmune process that had started during the immune response to live spirochetes ran its course in their absence. The blood test that Catherine took showed that she might have a hereditary risk for this type of Lyme arthritis (see Chapter 1).

While all parties to the treatment debate agree that antibiotic failures can occur with treatments of a month or less, the frequency of such failures is a matter of contention. Those physicians, governmental institutions, professional organizations, and public education groups recommending shorter treatment periods say that these failures are not so common that a blanket recommendation for longer therapy is justified. Those espousing longer treatments point to many patients in their practices or among their acquaintances who remain ill or relapse after receiving the treatments recommended in textbooks and professional periodicals. In many instances the public supporters of lengthier treatment schedules have personally experienced the persistence or remittance of illness. Only with longer treatments, sometimes involving the rotation or simultaneous use of more than one antibiotic, will cure be achieved, they argue. Even then, it is said, some cases may be incurable; the antibiotics serve only to keep the microorganisms in check. The theory advanced is that in many, not just a few, patients with chronic Lyme disease the spirochetes remain, perhaps hidden inside of cells, inaccessible to antibiotics.

Can these two different points of view be reconciled? At this time the answer is no, not completely. One reason is the difference in how Lyme disease is defined. The two groups may be talking about different groups of patients and therefore may be comparing "apples and oranges." From this perspective, both groups are right. If the respective definitions are accepted on their own terms, then a comparatively short treatment is sufficient for people with illnesses fitting the more restrictive definition, and longer treatment may be needed for some people whose illness meets the broader definition.

In the court of scientific opinion, at least, those who recommend the shorter treatment option present a more solid case. They have carried out controlled trials in which both the investigators and the patients were "blind" as to what medication the patients received. The other compelling feature of the case for limited treatment is that the definition of Lyme disease adopted for the studies was such that the patient groups would have included few if any patients who were not actually infected with *B. burgdorferi.* This is important, because if many such "pseudo-infections" are part of a study, then finding that antibiotics fall short of expectations would not be a surprise.

What the case for longer treatments may outwardly lack in scientific rigor is offset by the enthusiastic, almost evangelical commitment and passion of those believing it. These physicians and lay activists present numerous examples of people who fit their criteria for having Lyme disease and have failed to benefit from conventional treatment, and who have ultimately benefited from longer-term or even continuous antibiotic therapy. If there are people with a chronic, truly disabling illness that is relieved by long courses of oral or intravenous antibiotics, this is an important finding that ought to be considered when recommendations are made for medical treatment. After all, other chronic diseases, most prominently peptic ulcers, have been shown, quite unexpectedly, to be caused by bacteria. Within the broader definition of Lyme disease may be a disorder, possibly but not necessarily caused by *B. burgdorferi,* that is also treatable or manageable with antibiotics given for long periods (see Chapter 8). Until controlled trials with a control group receiving placebos are carried out on patients who have been diagnosed as having chronic Lyme disease using this broader definition, however, it is almost impossible to exhaustively assess the validity of these proposals. The impact of the placebo or nonspecific effect cannot be discounted. A collection of anecdotal accounts, as dramatic as they may sound, and as sincerely as they may be presented, is of limited value in the end. What these accounts of therapeutic success prompt is not a blanket change in treatment recommendations but controlled trials to see if all or part of the theory holds up. The federal government and large pharmaceutical companies have the resources to sponsor such a study; at least one such study, sponsored by the NIH, is planned.

Treatment of Lyme Disease during Pregnancy

Any infection during pregnancy brings with it anxiety over doing harm to the developing fetus, and Lyme disease is no exception. If the example of syphilis is taken as a guide, there would be reason to fear that Lyme disease would tragically be passed from mother to child in utero. Congenital syphilis and the irreparable damage it inflicted on countless unborn children was the principal reason that people were required to have a blood test for syphilis before marriage.

Happily, the odds of fetal death, congenital abnormalities, or infection at birth appear to be considerably lower for Lyme disease than for syphilis during pregnancy (see Chapter 1). By far the majority of human pregnancies complicated by a concurrent case of Lyme disease have been uneventful. If there is a risk of harmful fetal effects as a result of acute or chronic *B. burgdorferi* infections during pregnancy, then it appears to be too low to be readily detected.

Theoretically, the greatest risk of an untoward outcome is when a pregnancy is complicated by early Lyme disease. During early disease spirochetes are known to circulate in the blood and to be distributed to different organs, including, presumably, the placenta. A pregnancy occurring in a woman who has evidence of chronic Lyme disease or asymptomatic infection probably is not at any additional risk; people in this stage of disease seldom if ever have recoverable spirochetes in the blood. The tendency then is to regard only early infection in a pregnant woman as a special situation. Practically speaking, this means that if there is any clinical evidence of spread beyond the skin during early infection, the woman may be treated with an intravenous antibiotic. In any case—that is, for either acute or chronic disease—the tetracycline drugs are not used during pregnancy, because of the risk of harm to the teeth of the developing fetus.

Should Asymptomatic Infection Be Treated?

As the blood of more and more people is tested for Lyme disease, it is inevitable that individuals with no symptoms and signs compatible with active infection are found to be "seropositive." Such individuals may turn up when family members of a person with a confirmed case of Lyme disease are tested for evidence of *B. burgdorferi* infection. Sometimes entire communities are screened in public health assessments and epidemiologic surveys. Other populations that may be screened include laboratory researchers working with *B. burgdorferi*, veterinarians, and outdoor workers with a high risk of infection. If a Lyme disease vaccine becomes available (see Chapter 9), people may be tested to find out whether they already have been infected and thus are without need for the vaccine.

We need to ask what to do when someone who has no symptoms of Lyme disease is found, by whatever method, to be seropositive for the disease. As an example, let's say that during the course of a study of Lyme disease risk in outdoor workers, a healthy twenty-five-year-old forest ranger in New York is found to have both positive ELISA and positive Western blot test results for antibodies to *B. burgdorferi*. Under these circumstances it is very likely that the forest ranger had a *B. burgdorferi* infection in the past. But is the infection still present? Should he or she be treated with antibiotics? The answers to these questions are not known. There simply is not enough information to formulate a confident response. What is not known is, might an asymptomatic seropositive person develop chronic Lyme disease over the next five, ten, twenty, or forty years? and if this is possible, what is the likelihood of its occurring?

If a person is found either through screening or through individual testing to be seropositive, the individual should be asked about his or her symptoms. A problem with this approach is that many people have one or more of the less specific features of Lyme disease, and it may be hard to interpret the meaning of a report of fatigue, muscle aches, and occasional headache in an otherwise healthy person. It is likely that the constellation of these symptoms and a positive Lyme disease test is a coincidence. A next step might be to search more diligently for evidence of active infection in the body. But once the acute infection is over, it can be difficult to find the spirochetes in someone who is ill, much less in someone who is healthy. A quest for living bacteria in a healthy person may be just as futile with tomorrow's technology as it is with today's.

We are forced, then, to prophesy about the future using the meager data now available on Lyme disease. Our experience suggests—but by no means proves—that it would be very unlikely for the forest ranger to suffer chronic Lyme disease in the future. It's more likely that the infection occurred in the past and now is probably over, effectively eliminated by immunity. The residual is the telltale antibody response, which, incidentally, might protect the ranger against future *B. burgdorferi* infections. Lingering anxiety about the fate of the ranger and other asymptomatic seropositive persons is not entirely without justification, since our collective experience with other infectious diseases, notably AIDS, tuberculosis, and syphilis, has taught us to be concerned about diseases becoming symptomatic after having been asymptomatic for months or years.

AIDS, tuberculosis, and syphilis are characterized, like Lyme disease, by an acute infection that is followed years later by a chronic, disabling disease. The infected person may successfully subdue the initial inroads of the invading microorganism, but the invader persists, albeit quietly, hidden from the immune system. When the immune system's surveillance fails—that is, when it drops its guard—the AIDS virus, the tuberculosis bacillus, or the syphilis spirochete begins to proliferate again. Until that happens, though, the infected person may show no signs of illness. The only indication of past infection with one of these agents is a specific immune response. In the case of AIDS and syphilis, it is found in an antibody test; the immune response to tuberculosis is detected with a skin test. Not all asymptomatic persons go on to develop chronic diseases, but some do, and therefore accepted medical and public health policy holds that asymptomatic infection with these diseases should be identified and treated. This is done now with cases of asymptomatic tuberculosis and syphilis and undoubtedly will be done with HIV infection once a curative or otherwise preventative treatment is available.

There are two major differences between these three other infections and Lyme disease which give us cause to be optimistic about the destinies of untreated asymptomatic persons who at some time in the past were infected with *B. burgdorferi*. The first is that, unlike AIDS, tuberculosis, and syphilis, chronic Lyme disease is rarely fatal. The risk that a person seropositive for HIV infection will eventually die of AIDS is greater than 50 percent. The odds of having a fatal tuberculosis relapse or syphilis complication are lower but still substantial in comparison to the outcome with Lyme disease. Although some people with late Lyme disease do have permanent damage in spite of antibiotics, most respond to antibiotic therapy. There is a reasonable opportunity to reverse the process later, even if it is missed earlier. That may be small comfort to the person with lasting effects, but the risk of this happening must be weighed against the alternative: widespread screening for and treatment of silent infections.

The second reason for optimism is more speculative and is based on knowledge about the biology of these diseases. AIDS, tuberculosis, and syphilis are infections essentially only of humans. Their spread in the world depends on at least one human being transmitting the agent to another human being. The chances of this occurring are maximized if the infection persists for months to years. AIDS, tuberculosis, and syphilis achieve this. The late relapses and exacerbations serve to spread the microorganisms. But while humans are of pivotal importance for AIDS, tuberculosis, and syphilis, humans are unintentional and nonessential vessels for *B. burgdorferi* (see Chapter 3). If this spirochete depended on humans for its spread it would die off. Rodents and other small mammals are the real targets of *B. burgdorferi*. And in these animals, in fact, asymptomatic infections lasting weeks to months are common. Thus, the Lyme disease agent may be adapted for long-term survival in these other mammals but not in humans.

Antibiotic Therapy for Pets

There haven't been any controlled therapeutic trials of antibiotic treatments of dogs and other domestic animals with B. *burgdorferi* infection. Anecdotal evidence and extrapolation from the experience with humans and laboratory animals, however, suggest that tetracyclines, amoxicillin, and penicillin are generally effective treatments for B. *burgdorferi* infection in animals. Dogs are usually treated for less than a month with one of these oral antibiotics, but the optimal duration of therapy is unknown.

Other Conventional Treatments for Lyme Disease

So far we have been focusing exclusively on antibiotic treatments. Antibiotics are the cornerstone of treatment of Lyme disease, but additional measures may also be carried out. Some of the people whose stories we've followed throughout this book underwent these other kinds of treatments. Catherine, for example, received the anti-inflammatory agent hydroxychloroquine and ultimately had minor surgery, a synovectomy, to remove inflamed joint tissue. Roy had an artificial pacemaker temporarily placed in his heart. For someone such as Catherine, whose arthritis is unaffected by antibiotics, the other treatments become more important.

Whether they have early or late infection or the post–Lyme disease syndrome, some patients benefit from taking mild anti-inflammatory medicines for the joint and muscle aches and for headache. These medicines include aspirin and over-the-counter ibuprofen (Advil, Motrin, and other brand names) as well as similar drugs available by prescription. In some cases, more powerful drugs are used to resolve inflammation. One category of these more powerful drugs is commonly termed "steroids." These are related to but are not to be confused with the steroids associated with competitive sports; by *steroids,* physicians usually mean corticosteroids rather than the muscle-enhancing class of steroids. Hydrocortisone and prednisone are commonly prescribed forms of corticosteroids.

Prednisone and related medicines at one time constituted the only treatment for some cases of Lyme arthritis or neurologic disease, and some people seemed to respond to these agents alone. When antibiotics were discovered to be so beneficial for people with Lyme disease, however, corticosteroids were relegated to a supplementary role. Now they are sometimes used to treat people with heart involvement of Lyme disease, to speed return of their abnormal heartbeat to normal. Some physicians also prescribe a drug such as prednisone to relieve the pains and dysfunction of nervous system involvement by *B. burgdorferi*. The reasoning behind this approach to treatment is that the inflammation itself is producing damage, and that corticosteroids can limit this damage by reducing swelling and the number of cells in a critical area such as the heart, brain, or spinal cord. The other side of the coin, however, is that corticosteroids will also suppress the patient's immune response to some extent. A corticosteroid may serve to impair a person's own defenses against the spirochete. That is why, if corticosteroids are used, they are used only for a brief period, and only in conjunction with antibiotic treatment.

Alternative Medicines and Lyme Disease

The term *alternative medicines* has come to mean drugs and other treatments that have not usually had a place in the therapeutic armamentarium of modern Western medicine. Many alternative medicines trace their histories back for centuries, while others have been discovered more recently. The general public has always been interested in these alternative approaches to health care, and numerous people have made use of them. Recently, biomedical research agencies, including the National Institutes of Health, have shown more interest in exploring the therapeutic value of alternative medicines and have begun carrying out studies of their effects, including controlled clinical trials.

These evaluations likely will reveal which alternative medicines are effective, and why. Until then we are dependent for the most part on anecdotal reports. The argument is sometimes made that aspirin has become a widely used medicine without the benefit (or, some would say, the curse) of a controlled clinical trial. This is true, but there are many other examples of therapies that at one time were touted as providing a miraculous cure but subsequently were discredited after they were put to an unbiased test.

Like many other people with many other disabling illnesses, people who have been diagnosed with chronic Lyme disease have in their frustration looked to alternative medicines and therapies for relief. This may happen after one or more courses of antibiotics have had no effect, or only a temporary effect. Many of these alternative maneuvers, such as nutrition therapy and homeopathic medicines, are usually harmless to the person if not to his or her pocketbook. Other proposed treatments pose risks.

Perhaps the most startling and dangerous "alternative" proposal is that people who have chronic Lyme disease should be deliberately infected with the parasite that causes malaria. According to proponents of this procedure, the high body temperature that accompanies malaria infection would kill spirochetes in the body. They have pointed to the therapeutic application of this technique for syphilis of the nervous system before antibiotics became available. Although *B. burgdorferi* is slowed in its growth in the laboratory by temperatures just above normal body temperature, there is no evidence that a temporary fever will be effective in eliminating the spirochetes in a person. Moreover, there is considerable potential harm to the person from the treatment itself: the malaria parasite is obtained from the blood of another person, putting the recipient at risk of contracting other blood-borne diseases such as AIDS and hepatitis. The body temperature can be briefly raised more safely by hot water baths, but the effect is only transient; furthermore, this treatment puts elderly people and those with heart problems at risk of sudden death.

An equally radical if less hazardous therapy is injecting the currently available vaccine for dogs into people (Chapter 9). The reasoning behind this unapproved treatment is that, because they did not mount an effective immune response to the spirochetes to begin with, persons with chronic Lyme disease must have unresolved infections. Immunizing these people with the spirochetes, the theory goes, will boost the immune response. As was the case for the so-called malariotherapy, there might be a kernel of justification for such an approach.

Manipulating the immune system by immunization or some other technique may ultimately prove to be useful in treating Lyme disease and other chronic infections. But animal studies to date have shown that a simple immunization after infection has begun does not eliminate the infection. Much more experimental work needs to be done before it can be determined whether such a post-infection approach will be of benefit. Besides, the dog vaccine was designed for dogs, not people. There are components in it that have not been tested in people and that may be harmful for humans, especially if more than one immunization is carried out.

Use of a heavy metal to treat an infection is another new wrinkle on an old practice. At least one practitioner espouses the use of a silver compound to treat people said to have chronic Lyme disease. Mercury, antimony, and arsenic chemicals have been used in the past as therapy for infection, but this was before antibiotics or other safer therapeutic agents became available. If the silver or other metal compounds benefit some patients with chronic Lyme disease, it is as likely due to an anti-inflammatory effect as an antibacterial effect.

Another novel but still unproven therapy is the attempt to boost the infected person's immune response to B. burgdorferi by administering what has been called "transfer factor." This is an as-yet-undefined substance or substances produced in a successful defense against an infection. It is then passed on to another person or animal to aid in the battle. In the case of Lyme disease, the transfer factor is said to be in the milk produced by cows that have been vaccinated with B. burgdorferi cells.

Finally, if someone is pursuing alternative treatments for Lyme disease instead of, rather than in addition to, traditional treatments, that person may be missing the chance to get effective, proven treatment. The best recommendation for someone with Lyme disease is to get antibiotic treatment from a licensed professional. Such a professional can also be a good source of advice about potentially harmful, ineffective, and costly alternative treatments.

Conclusions

As has been evident through this chapter, Lyme disease has more than the usual share of controversies and conflicting claims. Yes, there are differences in how Lyme disease, especially in its chronic form, is defined. And yes, the choices for treatment are wide, ranging from a couple of weeks of oral antibiotics to several months of intravenous therapy.

On what basis should physicians and patients make treatment decisions, especially when they know that a commonly perceived consequence of antibiotic failure is a life of joint pains and mental dysfunction, as well as such other complaints as tiring easily? The available evidence from scientifically based studies does not provide all the answers by any means, but it does provide some. The studies show that the currently recommended oral antibiotic treatments of two to four weeks for early Lyme disease are effective. Certainly they are as effective as antibiotic therapies for other common infections, such as strep throat, urinary tract infection, and gonorrhea, about which there is nowhere near this kind of controversy. The present evidence also shows that giving additional antibiotics, at least in courses of conventional length, seldom provides sustained relief to people with the post–Lyme disease syndrome.

There is a subset of people with the diagnosis of chronic Lyme disease whose symptoms do respond to antibiotic treatments lasting two months or longer. However, this phenomenon, as important as it might be for certain people's health and for our concepts about infections, has not been adequately studied. Neither side of the controversy can conclusively say whether or not the perceived benefit of long-term antibiotics for this condition is derived from the killing of spirochetes by antibiotics, from nonspecific actions of antibiotics, or from the placebo effect—or is simply the result of the passage of time.

A conservative estimate is that in more than half the cases of late Lyme disease in which the major manifestation is arthritis with joint swelling, abnormal neurologic function, or long-lasting skin inflammation (acrodermatitis chronica atrophicans) there is improvement with a single course of antibiotics, administered for about a month if given by mouth or for two to four weeks if given intravenously.

8

If It Isn't Lyme Disease, What Is It?

■ Evelyn and Tad and their two young children had lived in their new home just outside of San Francisco for two months when Evelyn's illness began. A literary agent in the city, Evelyn thrived on hectic workdays and physically active weekends, playing tennis when she and Tad were not fixing up their Victorian era house. Then, in the last week of October, Evelyn came down with what she thought was the flu. Her muscles ached, and for a few days she felt too feverish and weak to get out of bed. The fever subsided after a few days, but she could not, as she said, "keep up the pace" she was accustomed to.

Months later Evelyn still barely made it through a day at work without feeling drained. Although she went to bed earlier than usual, her sleep was fitful and she did not feel refreshed in the morning. On Saturdays and Sundays she napped to try to catch up on her sleep. Her joints hurt (but they weren't swollen), and her muscles felt stiff and sore in the morning. Twitches in her legs occasionally bothered her, and her throat hurt. Although her temperature never rose above 100°F, she sometimes felt chilled. Evelyn wasn't aware of eating more than usual, but her weight had increased by ten pounds over the last several months.

Evelyn's grandfather had developed Alzheimer's disease late in life, and she secretly feared that she had the same condition. She was concerned because she was becoming increasingly forgetful and was having difficulty concentrating. Also, sometimes she had to retrace her steps to remember why she had gone from one room into another. An avid reader in the past, she now had difficulty following the story line of a novel. And she sometimes could not come up with the right word when conversing or making a presentation at work.

Tad was very supportive at first. He reassured Evelyn that she would soon bounce back and that she ought to think positively instead of brooding over her problems. Still, he was feeling more and more stress himself. He was taking on more of the housework, including most of the cooking at night. The decreased frequency of their lovemaking concerned him, too.

Evelyn had already been to two physicians. Her gynecologist, who was her primary care physician, saw her first. To get another opinion about Evelyn's case, the gynecologist asked an internist to see her "in consultation." Although she was usually articulate, Evelyn found it difficult to explain what she was experiencing. It was easier and less embarrassing for her to talk about the fatigue and the joint pains than about the difficulty she was having in concentrating and remembering. After doing a physical exam and routine laboratory tests, the gynecologist reassured her that she did not have cancer or anemia. The internist then ordered x-rays of joints and additional blood tests, including those relating to thyroid and adrenal gland function, and tests for autoimmune diseases such as lupus and rheumatoid arthritis. There was no evidence of arthritis in the x-ray films, and the only blood test abnormality found was a slightly elevated cholesterol level. The internist counseled Evelyn about a low-fat diet and told her that she was in otherwise good health.

For a few days after that appointment Evelyn felt better, knowing that she did not have anything serious wrong with her, and she resolved to get back to her old pace by the end of the month. Both Tad and Evelyn were discouraged, though, when she was unable to do this. The aching joints and fatigue were as bothersome as ever; and now Evelyn began having recurrent headaches, and sometimes dropped things she was holding, such as silverware. She returned to the internist and told him more about the changes in her mental functioning. His physical examination again was unrevealing, but he said he was concerned about Evelyn's symptoms, and for this reason he ordered an *MRI scan,* a computer-assisted viewing (like an x-ray) of the entire brain. This was interpreted as normal, as was an *electromyogram,* a test of her muscles and nerves. By that time the results of more specialized blood tests that the physician had ordered were in. Everything was negative except the Lyme disease ELISA result. This was reported by the testing laboratory as being positive.

Saying, "Now we have something to treat," the physician prescribed a two-week treatment with ceftriaxone, which was given by vein at home. After the first few days of the antibiotics Evelyn began to feel somewhat stronger and could do more around the house, and by the time the treatments stopped she was determined to return to work full time. Within two weeks, however, she felt as tired as ever, and she still had aching joints. She resumed taking intravenous antibiotics, this time cefotaxime, which she took for an entire month. Evelyn and Tad ended up paying for the last two weeks of therapy out of their savings, because the insurance company would not reimburse them for more than the first two weeks. For a time they thought it was worth it, because for the first two weeks of therapy her condition partially improved. But by the last week of treatment Evelyn and her husband were not sure any more: her symptoms had begun to worsen again.

At that point the internist consulted an infectious disease specialist, who suggested that the Lyme disease ELISA test be repeated. The second ELISA test was also positive, but the follow-up Western blot was reported as negative. On the basis of these results, the infectious disease specialist said that he doubted whether Evelyn had ever had Lyme disease. Evelyn's physicians told her that if she had Lyme disease she should have responded to treatment by now. They reassured Evelyn and her husband that she was not infected and recommended that she see a psychiatrist because she seemed depressed and anxious. Evelyn angrily replied: "I know I'm depressed and anxious, but it's because of my physical illness and not because I'm crazy to start with." Leaving the office, she added, "I *know* that it's real!"

A Diagnostic Dilemma

This is a discouraging story for Evelyn, her husband, and her physicians, and one repeated with different variations many times every day throughout the country. Men as well as women, older people and younger, have had similar experiences. The illness may begin suddenly, as in Evelyn's case, or start more insidiously. Commonly reported symptoms are tiring easily, failing to get refreshing sleep, and experiencing joint aches, painful muscles and connective tissues, and sluggish thinking.

Did Evelyn have Lyme disease? Some physicians and others would say that she did, that the infection was still active, and that she needed to be back on antibiotics to get sustained improvement. Others would answer no, and moreover, would say that the intravenous treatment was a waste of time and money. This more skeptical group would also argue that the weeks of antibiotics put Evelyn at risk of side effects, some of them serious. A third group of physicians might concede that Evelyn had been infected with *Borrelia burgdorferi* at some time in the past, but would caution that her current symptoms could not be accounted for by active infection.

Who is correct? It depends on how "Lyme disease" is defined. Those holding a broadly inclusive set of criteria might point out that Evelyn lived in an area, northern California, where Lyme disease has been reported and that her symptoms of prolonged fatigue, joint pains, and mild disturbances of intellectual function can occur in that disease. They might go on to say that both the positive Lyme disease test ELISA and the temporary responses to antibiotic treatment were evidence of *B. burgdorferi* infection.

Those with a more restricted definition might respond that Evelyn did not have an illness that met the criteria of the diagnosis of Lyme disease. They would acknowledge that transmission of *B. burgdorferi* to humans in northern California has been documented, but they would say that the risk of disease is many times lower there than in many areas of the Northeast. Furthermore, nothing in Evelyn's history suggests that she was exposed to ticks, and she did not have a rash compatible with erythema migrans. And she had neither true arthritis nor a neurologic disorder, such as facial weakness, which would be more typical of Lyme disease. Although the ELISA test was positive, the Western blot was not. In these experts' view, Evelyn's ELISA result was likely a false-positive reaction.

Because there are two views of what can be included under the label "chronic Lyme disease," we need a way to distinguish between the two definitions. The more restrictive definition requires either (1) the occurrence of erythema migrans before onset of chronic manifestations; or (2) involvement of a specific organ (such as the nervous system, the heart, or a joint) and laboratory evidence of infection. The latter would be ELISA and Western blot test results showing the presence of antibodies to *B. burgdorferi*, or direct detection of the microorganism in the person. Moreover, the person would need to have been in an area in which there is a risk of *B. burgdorferi* infection. A stay-at-home in the Fiji Islands could not have Lyme disease; a resident of New Jersey or Germany might. Inasmuch as these more restrictive criteria constitute the definition used in most medical reference books, I reserve use of the term *chronic Lyme disease* for cases of illness meeting this definition.

As stated, some physicians and Lyme disease researchers accept a less stringent definition of chronic Lyme disease. Symptoms that cannot be easily localized to a certain organ or body system are prominent in their criteria. These symptoms include fatigue, generalized aches and pains, poor sleep, and problems in concentration and memory (described as a "mental fog" by some patients). Published as well as informally distributed lists of compatible symptoms have also named such problems as an altered ability to smell and taste, irritability and impulsive behavior, headache, and frequent colds. At one time or another most of the population has experienced at least one of these many symptoms. Oftentimes a diagnosis is made in the absence of traditional laboratory evidence of *B. burgdorferi* infection or a history compatible with exposure to the tick vector, the arguments being that the current tests are insensitive and that Lyme disease is more widespread than is appreciated. When I use this looser, less rigorous view of long-lasting Lyme disease I call it "chronic Lyme disease, broadly defined."

If, in her physicians' opinion, Evelyn did not have active Lyme disease, what did she have? It is easier to identify what she did not have than what she did have. The directions in which and the lengths to which the answer is pursued depend on the physician's interests and his or her level of comfort with being uncertain about diagnosis. A public health official counting cases of Lyme disease in California might care little, on a professional level at least, about what Evelyn really had as long as her illness did not meet the current case definition for Lyme disease; this official would only want to know whether or not to include Evelyn in the tally of cases.

The infectious disease specialist who is oriented to what antibiotics have to offer the patient might feel similarly: in the absence of evidence of infection, there is little more that such a specialist can do. The diagnosis that he or she might use instead is *chronic fatigue syndrome* (this syndrome is discussed later in this chapter).

As happened with Evelyn, a "not guilty" verdict with regard to Lyme disease is often followed by a referral to another medical specialist. A rheumatologist—a specialist in joint, connective tissue, and immunologic diseases—might carry out additional blood tests in an effort to detect more subtle abnormalities in the immune system or skeleton. Failing to find such an abnormality, the rheumatologist might conclude that Evelyn has *fibromyalgia* (also discussed below). A neurologist (a specialist in diseases of the brain) might evaluate Evelyn for early evidence of a dementing condition such as Alzheimer's disease. There are tests and procedures for determining whether a person has such a condition. A psychiatrist, who is often consulted only after other possibilities have been exhausted, might explore with Evelyn whether she was depressed or for some other reason had a disordered sleep pattern.

The physician who referred Evelyn to the psychiatrist might have said something like this: "We looked for an organic cause but could not find any, so the problem must be functional." This means that they had looked for certain known diseases ("organic causes") and, failing to find one, had concluded that there really was nothing wrong with Evelyn's organs or tissues. In other words, he thought the problem was a behavioral, or a "functional," one. The consulting psychiatrist indeed might explore this possibility and might even conclude that Evelyn could benefit from psychotherapy. Perhaps there was a deep-seated reason for what could be interpreted as a withdrawal from work and family. There are at least two other outcomes from the visit to the psychiatrist. He or she might diagnose Evelyn's illness as an atypical form of depression, which is just as much an "organic" disorder as asthma or high blood pressure is. Or the consulting psychiatrist might agree with Evelyn that her primary problem was a medical illness, after all, and that the depression, anxiety, or sleep disorder were secondary responses.

A patient who has seen a variety of specialists and who by now is confused and frustrated returns to the internist or family practitioner with heavy medical chart in hand.

Is "Lyme Disease" Equivalent to "*Borrelia Burgdorferi* Infection"?

Before reconsidering Evelyn's diagnosis, let's back up to the point when her physicians concluded that she did *not* have Lyme disease. As should be clear by now, such a conclusion is controversial. Some of these differences of opinion over diagnosis and management lie in the fact that some people distinguish between "Lyme disease" and *B. burgdorferi* infection. Separated in many people's minds are, on the one hand, a clinical syndrome, "Lyme disease," which might be defined on the basis of symptoms in a way that is valid and useful for patient care, and, on the other hand, an infection by a particular microorganism, *B. burgdorferi*.

The acknowledged difficulty in detecting the microorganism widens the gulf between the concepts of Lyme disease and a spirochete infection. In situations such as this—that is, when the diagnostic line between infection and no infection is fuzzy—it is tempting to make a diagnosis on the basis of a constellation of symptoms alone rather than a more comprehensive view incorporating not only symptoms but also laboratory data and the likelihood of becoming infected. Attributing a frustrating, disabling, and chronic disease to a potentially treatable infection is appealing for both physician and patient. Nevertheless, diagnosis on these grounds may be hasty: there may be other explanations for Evelyn's illness.

To invoke one type of bacterium to account for all cases of what falls under a broader diagnostic umbrella of "Lyme disease" is akin to saying that all or most forms of arthritis of the knee are due to *B. burgdorferi*. There are many kinds of arthritis, only one of which is Lyme arthritis. A common form of arthritis, rheumatoid arthritis, *may* be initiated by one or more infectious agents, but this has not been proven. Even the suspicion that an infection is the causative agent has not yet led to a widely accepted treatment or a means of prevention.

Those physicians holding a more restricted definition of chronic Lyme disease appear to be on the firmest scientific ground, to judge from the medical literature and textbooks. But this is not to say that the observations of those arguing for a more broadly defined chronic Lyme disease are invalid. If, as has been suggested by some, certain patients do benefit from extended courses of therapy and only approach normal health while being treated with antibiotics, then these reports warrant serious consideration. As has been discussed, this positive outcome with antibiotics may be the consequence of a placebo effect, either of the medication itself or of the physician's optimism and encouragement. Alternatively, nonspecific effects of antibiotics may play a role in producing the patient's sense of greater well-being—perhaps through their as yet poorly understood anti-inflammatory actions (see Chapter 6). Nevertheless, until a group of patients meeting the broader definition of Lyme disease are treated "blindly" and randomly in a controlled trial, it may be short-sighted to reject out-of-hand some of these reports of inexplicable benefits from antibiotics.

Thousands of people have been treated as if they had Lyme disease. Many of those responding to antibiotics did not have what has traditionally been accepted as evidence of *B. burgdorferi* infection. Perhaps some of these people had infections with *B. burgdorferi* that were less obvious. Perhaps some of them had chronic infections with other bacteria, known or unknown. Perhaps there is no benefit from antibiotics in these circumstances other than their placebo and nonspecific effects. Some people have developed serious reactions to or complications from treatment of what was thought to be Lyme disease. This controversy is not trivial. It affects the health, well-being, and pocketbooks of many people, and it needs to be resolved.

The Need to Diagnose and Be Diagnosed

Instead of Lyme disease, Evelyn might have any of the diseases described below. We may be allotting more space to a discussion of these diagnoses than is merited considering how infrequently some of them affect people. The truth is that many human ills do not conveniently fall into one diagnostic pigeonhole or another. Some illnesses find their place when a new diagnosis, such as chronic fatigue syndrome or fibromyalgia, gains acceptance. Many other illnesses continue to be rather less specific and not easily categorized.

Both the physician and the patient would prefer it if the illness fit into a diagnostic category, even if the illness is square and the hole is round. By training and personality, most physicians are more comfortable and confident when they can provide a diagnosis of this or that disease. And patients often prefer any diagnosis to no diagnosis at all. A known diagnosis, even if grave, may be feared less than the unknown and its attendant uncertainty. Upon hearing a diagnosis of terminal cancer or AIDS, a person may, paradoxically, say, "What a relief it is to find out for sure."

If some people are comforted even by hearing a diagnosis of a life-threatening or stigmatized disease, imagine the greater acceptance of a diagnosis that identifies the patient's disease as one that is curable and stigma-free. Lyme disease is such a disease. The effective treatments are nonthreatening antibiotics, not medicines that make one's face puffy, one's hair fall out, one's blood count drop, or one's penis become inopportunely flaccid. Lyme disease is a disorder primarily (but not exclusively) of the middle and upper classes of developed countries, not of an economic underclass or of developing countries. It is acquired as a result of what are viewed as healthful and admirable activities: working in the garden, playing out of doors, in the grass, and hiking or hunting in the forest, among other things. For some eternal optimists, it may even be viewed as a diagnosis of some social currency. After all, some famous people have freely talked about their Lyme disease to the mass media.

Lyme disease is not the first disorder to be fashionable in this way, nor is it likely to be the last. The need of physicians and patients to find a mutually acceptable diagnosis is such that other real or imagined conditions have been named as the cause of otherwise inexplicable illnesses. The history of medicine records many of these. An apt example of this phenomenon from an earlier part of the twentieth century is chronic brucellosis, which, although not well publicized, was the "Lyme disease" of its day in the United States. Brucellosis itself is a serious infection that people inadvertently acquire from drinking unpasteurized milk or having direct contact with cows, goats, or pigs. Dairy workers, ranchers, veterinarians, and slaughterhouse workers are at the highest risk for brucellosis. The infection is caused by the *Brucella* group of bacteria, which can be detected in the blood and certain tissues of acutely ill patients. As the infection evolves into a more chronic, persistent form, it becomes harder to diagnose by the direct isolation of organisms. In this case the history, the physical exam, and a laboratory test for antibodies to *Brucella* become important to the diagnosis. (Does this sound familiar?) The antibody test for *Brucella* was probably neither better nor worse than the current assays for antibodies to *B. burgdorferi*. In both tests cross-reactive antibodies arising from other infections can result in false-positive results.

When an astute physician combined a convincing story of risk factors, compatible symptoms and physical signs, and a finding in the blood of high levels of *Brucella* antibodies, the diagnosis of chronic brucellosis was usually accurate. The definition of chronic brucellosis, however, was broadened by some physicians to include illnesses that today might be just as easily diagnosed as chronic Lyme disease, broadly defined. Fatigue, chilliness, mental lethargy, and muscle and joint aches were sufficient to elicit suspicion of chronic brucellosis. Blood was drawn and sent off for the *Brucella* antibody test. The criteria for a diagnosis were relaxed to include lower levels of antibodies. Such laboratory results were less reliably predictive of true infection, especially if the risk of infection was low to begin with.

The inappropriate use of the term *chronic brucellosis* for other disorders was eventually exposed, and the diagnosis fell out of favor—but not before many patients were given and accepted the diagnosis. Many of these people were treated with antibiotics, some for long periods of time. And enough of them responded with symptomatic improvement that the diagnosis of chronic brucellosis remained a popular diagnosis in some regions for years.

What did these people actually have? The question could just as easily be, If it isn't Lyme disease, what is it? There will remain many people whose disability or illness cannot be categorized. Their conditions do not meet the textbook criteria for any of the diseases named in the insurance company manual or governmental listings. Does that mean that they do not have a "real" illness, that it is "all in their mind," or that they cannot be helped? The answer is no to each question. What they and their physicians may have to live with, though, is a degree of uncertainty about the diagnosis. The focus should be not on what the illness is, but on how to help the patient feel better.

Uncertain Definitions Lead to Uncertain Diagnoses

A disease can be placed somewhere between two poles. At one pole is a disorder unambiguously defined by the presence of a microorganism, by a certain mutation, or by a specific pathologic change in an organ. Examples of such diseases are measles, Down's syndrome, and breast cancer. A child with the measles virus in his body will be ill with the disease measles. A newborn baby whose cells have three of chromosome number 21 instead of the usual two will show the signs of Down's syndrome. A woman whose biopsy under the microscope has the telltale signs of malignant change has breast cancer.

At the other pole is a disease defined only by the patient's subjective symptoms, perhaps supplemented by the physician's observations. Migraine headache is usually diagnosed on the basis of a person's description of his or her headache attacks and the events leading up to them. Depression, panic attacks, and obsessive-compulsive disorder are some of the many psychiatric disorders whose diagnosis depends to a large extent on the patient's story and his or her responses to questions. There is not yet—and may never be—an infallible lab test for these conditions.

Most medical disorders, however, fall somewhere between these two poles. A peptic ulcer disease may be diagnosed on the basis of symptoms alone, but there is more certainty if the gastroenterologist looks through a flexible tube and sees an ulcer or two just beyond the stomach. Likewise, a patient in the emergency room may tell a story that is characteristic of a heart attack and be rushed to the cardiac care unit on that basis. But if the story varies from the typical, then physicians depend more on the electrocardiogram and the measurement of certain enzymes in the blood for diagnosis. They may even need to take a special x-ray of the heart to look for blockage of the arteries.

At this point in time Lyme disease is closer to the subjective, symptom-based pole than to the objective, pathology-based pole. Until better laboratory tests, such as the PCR assay, become widely available, diagnosis rests principally and appropriately on the patient's history. A laboratory test for antibodies can be helpful, but it is not the be-all and end-all of diagnosis. Most patients' diagnoses of Lyme disease have not depended on the recovery of *B. burgdorferi* from blood, skin, or other organs, either.

Many of the disorders confused with broadly defined chronic Lyme disease are also diagnosed principally on the basis of symptoms. The sets of symptoms defining these diseases overlap to greater or lesser extents. Without a hallmark or otherwise unique signature for each disease—excepting the occasional isolation of *B. burgdorferi* from the patient—it is difficult to know precisely what is going on. Is it Lyme disease or fibromyalgia? Is it chronic fatigue syndrome or depression? Obviously it is important to know whether someone has an active infection with *B. burgdorferi,* because antibiotics are without question the appropriate therapy. But if active infection can be ruled out, then the remaining possibilities have common as well as distinguishing aspects. Even if the physician cannot be sure whether a person has chronic fatigue syndrome or depression, post-infection syndrome or fibromyalgia, the lack of a firm diagnosis does not mean that nothing can be done, since some of the same therapeutic approaches are used to treat each of these disorders. What works for depression may also be effective to some extent for cases of chronic fatigue syndrome and fibromyalgia. Uncertainty about the illness's pigeonhole does not imply helplessness.

Diagnoses That Should Not Be Overlooked

Before considering those disorders, such as fibromyalgia, that are most commonly taken for broadly defined chronic Lyme disease (and vice versa), the physician may try to rule out, or exclude from the list of diagnostic possibilities, some conditions that it would be unfortunate to miss. Some of these diseases are treatable if caught early enough. Others are not necessarily treatable—in the sense that the patient can be cured—but the disease's progress can be slowed, halted, or partially reversed by medications. The opportunity for early diagnosis may be missed if the physician mistakenly thinks that the patient has Lyme disease and neglects other possibilities for too long.

An example of a communicable disease that might be confused with chronic Lyme disease is infection with HIV, the virus that causes AIDS. Before developing characteristic AIDS, an HIV-infected person may suffer from easy fatigability, headache, muscle aches, and other nonspecific symptoms. In this situation an ELISA test and follow-up Western blot test for antibodies should reveal the presence of antibodies to HIV. Testing for HIV antibodies is recommended for evaluation of cases of unexplained chronic fatigue syndrome. For the same reasons, this test is an important part of the evaluation of some patients suspected to have chronic Lyme disease. Delay in the start of preventive treatment of HIV-infected persons can result in increased hospitalizations and early mortality.

Syphilis can cause nervous system disorders that are like those of Lyme disease. Patients with syphilis also frequently have false-positive ELISA tests, because the syphilis spirochete and *B. burgdorferi* have much in common. The two infections can be distinguished from each other with another antibody test, which over the years has gone by several names (two in current use are "RPR" and "VDRL"). This antibody test is usually positive in syphilis and negative in Lyme disease.

Other infectious diseases that may manifest as excessive fatigue and unrefreshing sleep are infectious mononucleosis, better known as "mono"; toxoplasmosis, a common parasitic disease acquired by having contact with cat feces or consuming inadequately cooked beef; viral hepatitis without yellow jaundice; and tuberculosis. Hepatitis would be detected, even if not suspected initially, by routine blood tests that check the function of the liver. The other infections would require another test or two for confirmation of the diagnosis. In the case of tuberculosis, the next diagnostic step would be a skin test and possibly a chest x-ray.

Cancers, like infections, should not be overlooked. Chronic Lyme disease is not commonly confused with cancer, but if it were to be, the consequences of delayed diagnosis would be great. Most people would not think of Lyme disease if they began to cough up blood, felt a new lump in their neck or breast, or had severe pains in their abdomen. But they might consider it, even believe it, if the cancer's presence early on was signaled by a sense of fatigue, a low-grade fever, and some muscle aches. Of course, in an early stage cancer might not be readily identified even if suspected. But sticking to a diagnosis of Lyme disease when reliable laboratory tests do not confirm its presence and antibiotics have not produced a cure needlessly delays the performance of a thorough search for the real cause of the illness.

Instead of cancer, the cause may be an autoimmune disease, such as lupus erythematosus or rheumatoid arthritis. Most forms of these latter disorders have their own distinctive symptoms and thus are not usually confused with chronic Lyme disease. A person with rheumatoid arthritis, for example, may have a swollen, painful knee joint, as someone with Lyme disease might have. But the smaller joints of the hands and feet are also usually involved in rheumatoid arthritis; this would be less common in Lyme arthritis. If the person's symptoms and signs are suggestive of Lyme disease but may be due to an autoimmune disease, specific laboratory tests may be done to identify or rule out abnormalities that are associated with different varieties of autoimmune diseases but not with Lyme disease. Most people with rheumatoid arthritis have in their blood unique antibodies called *rheumatoid factor;* some patients with Lyme arthritis have rheumatoid factor in their blood, too, but at concentrations that are undetectable by the standard assay. To test for systemic lupus erythematosus and certain other autoimmune diseases, an assay for *antinuclear antibodies* is performed. Another commonly performed blood test that indicates the presence not only of autoimmune disease but also of some cancers and infections is the *erythrocyte sedimentation rate,* often called an "ESR" or "sed rate." The higher the rate, the less likely it is that the patient's disorder is Lyme disease.

There are several treatments for autoimmune disease, but many have in common the goal of suppressing the immune system until the harmful responses a patient makes against herself or himself are controlled. Examples are methotrexate, azathioprine (Imuran), and corticosteroid drugs such as prednisone. Antibiotics do not have these powerful immunosuppressive effects. Although infectious agents are suspected of being a stimulus or trigger for some autoimmune diseases, there has been little convincing evidence to date that antibiotics are useful in treating these conditions after they have developed. Thus, there may be more to lose than to gain by prescribing prolonged antibiotic treatment of a person who instead of the suspected *B. burgdorferi* infection actually has rheumatoid arthritis or another autoimmune disease.

Allergies, too, are an abnormal immune response, but instead of reacting inappropriately against himself or herself, the person with allergies reacts inappropriately to substances in the environment. The reactions are said to be inappropriate because they probably are not helpful to the allergic person—that is, there is unlikely to be an advantage to being hypersensitive to cat hair, house dust, or goldenrod pollen. Unlike drug allergies, these environmental stimuli are liable to cause respiratory symptoms rather than a rash. But many people undergoing a period of heightened allergic reactions report some Lyme disease symptoms; they may have prominent fatigue, a generalized achiness, and slowed thinking in addition to their watery eyes, runny nose, and wheezing. Many people with allergies and these more nonspecific symptoms benefit when the allergic reactions are controlled with medications or desensitization with so-called allergy shots.

Multiple sclerosis is a disabling and eventually fatal disease of young and middle-aged adults which may in some of its features resemble chronic Lyme disease of the nervous system. Like Lyme disease, MS can affect different parts of the nervous system at the same time and can wax and wane in intensity. Fatigue is a common complaint in both multiple sclerosis and chronic Lyme disease. Although most people with multiple sclerosis have a characteristic pattern of findings on laboratory tests of the cerebrospinal fluid and MRI scans of the brain, some people in the early stages of MS may be difficult to diagnose conclusively. Because multiple sclerosis is less readily controlled with medication than certain forms of cancer and autoimmune disease, delayed diagnosis may not necessarily have a tragic outcome. What more commonly happens is that a person suspected of having MS holds on to the hope that the deteriorating condition is due to *B. burgdorferi* infection and not to the fitful but inexorable thinning of the nerves that is MS.

People with MS who have this chance of cure in mind may even undergo antibiotic treatment. If a temporary, natural remission of MS coincides with the antibiotic therapy, these patients and their families may attribute their improvement to that therapy. Anecdotes of such improvements have been publicized, and, understandably, they have a great impact on patients and their families and prompt others to seek such cures. But while multiple sclerosis is another autoimmune-type disease whose beginning may be traced to a poorly resolved infection, there is little compelling evidence that active infection with *B. burgdorferi* or any another bacterium is the culprit. Thus, antibiotics would not be expected to benefit someone with MS, and their use is futile under these conditions. These aspects of multiple sclerosis may also be seen in amyotrophic lateral sclerosis, popularly known as Lou Gehrig's disease.

Endocrine, hormonal, and metabolic disorders are another group of diseases that may in some ways resemble broadly defined chronic Lyme disease. A person with undiagnosed diabetes may feel inordinately fatigued, or may have pains and tingling sensations in the arms and legs which resemble Lyme disease of the nervous system. The routine blood tests and urinalysis that Evelyn had when she was first seen would likely have detected diabetes that was severe enough to be producing these symptoms. In these tests, excessively high levels of glucose, a simple sugar, would suggest diabetes.

The other endocrine systems that are commonly checked in these circumstances are the thyroid and adrenal glands. Under- or overactivity of the thyroid gland in the neck can lead to fatigue and other general symptoms. When the adrenal gland, which produces cortisone and related hormones, is not functioning properly, the result is usually weakness and tiredness. There are simple blood tests for these thyroid and adrenal disorders, but they are not usually part of the package of tests that patients have when they enter the hospital or have a routine physical exam. The physician has to include thyroid disease or adrenal disorders in the differential diagnosis (the list of possible causes of the patient's symptoms) and specifically request these tests.

Fibromyalgia and Chronic Fatigue Syndrome

If you were to look in the table of contents of an old medical textbook, you would not find a listing for fibromyalgia or chronic fatigue syndrome. That's not to say these conditions are new under the sun, however. These older textbooks described other conditions, such as "fibrositis," which had many of the features of fibromyalgia, and "neurasthenia," whose symptoms were similar to those of what is today called chronic fatigue syndrome (CFS). (Another diagnosis that is not as popular as it once was is chronic brucellosis, described earlier in this chapter.) At the turn of the century neurasthenia, commonly considered a disease of "brain workers" and the consequence of "nervous exhaustion," affected several famous or soon-to-be-famous writers, artists, politicians, and other leaders of the day. The flowering of health spas at such places as Battle Creek, Michigan, occurred at the same time that the number of diagnoses of neurasthenia and related disorders was increasing. The prescribed cure for neurasthenia was mental rest and physical exercise.

Like both neurasthenia and fibrositis, fibromyalgia and CFS are located close to, if not precisely at, the subjective extreme of the spectrum of diagnosis. The patient's symptoms or his or her responses to the physician's questions form the principal basis for diagnosis. There are few laboratory or other procedural tests that support these diagnoses, let alone confirm them. Certainly, there is nothing to date like the antibody test for *B. burgdorferi* infection. Because their symptoms overlap those for chronic Lyme disease, especially as it is broadly defined, fibromyalgia and CFS may be confused with that disorder, as well as with each other. Further complicating the picture is the role of *B. burgdorferi* infection in apparently initiating some cases of fibromyalgia or CFS. Some cases of undisputed Lyme disease have been followed by illnesses consistent with fibromyalgia or CFS.

The similarities between fibromyalgia, CFS, and what has been called the post–Lyme disease syndrome have been pointed out. How *B. burgdorferi* initiates CFS and fibromyalgia is not known; it may be that the immune, endocrine, and nervous systems wage an inappropriately prolonged fight against the infection. The anti-infection machine has been switched on, so to speak, but the usually reliable automatic turn-off switch does not function at the right time, and the machine continues to operate. What is of benefit for a human or an animal fighting an infection, such as the urge to rest in order to recuperate, becomes over time the symptom of easy fatigability—and this can become quite a liability if a person has a family and job to attend to.

Although fibromyalgia and CFS are sometimes considered to have been provoked by a case of Lyme disease, these conditions are usually not associated with a prior *B. burgdorferi* infection. Most experts on CFS think that this condition may be the final common pathway after an encounter or experience with a number of different agents and stressors, most likely infections of one sort or another. Several known microorganisms have been implicated, but none stands out as the obvious cause of most cases of CFS. The disorder may be incited by a virus or bacterium that has not yet been discovered and named, despite the fact that the search for this hypothetical microorganism has been intense.

For some people the cause of CFS may not be an infectious organism at all. Exposure to a chemical or another kind of toxin has also been blamed, most notably in the case of sick building syndrome and the Gulf War syndrome (described below). It is conceivable that the origin of these disorders lies not outside a person but inside. A prolonged period of stress, caused perhaps by a divorce or the loss of a job, is in many respects the bodily equivalent of an acute infection. Many of the same physiologic responses that occur with an infection also occur with stress or bereavement. If a poorly regulated response to infection can cause CFS or fibromyalgia, why not an unregulated response to stress? The stress may due to changes in a person's life, to a primary psychiatric disorder, such as depression, or to a combination of the two. Ironically, turn-of-the-century proponents of the concept of neurasthenia saw the disorder as a response to social stresses and internal "nervous" stresses, what we today call "burn out." In our time a foreign invader, such as a virus or bacterium, or a toxic substance, such as a pesticide or fumes from an oil-field fire, finds greater acceptance than stress as a cause of disorders like neurasthenia. Somehow, being a victim of a microorganism or environmental contaminant is an easier cross to bear than our own human frailty in a complicated society.

Like Lyme disease, CFS and fibromyalgia are diagnosed using strict criteria that have been agreed upon by physicians and other experts. These diagnostic criteria were designed primarily for studying the epidemiology of the diseases. Epidemiology is the science of disorders in populations: changes in their frequency over time and in different locations and groups of people. Epidemiologic studies are valuable for tracking the spread of disease and for identifying who is at risk of disease. If these studies are to be reliable and reproducible, strict case definitions, upon which most investigators agree, are needed.

The experimental reasoning applied in epidemiologic studies is that it is better to err in the direction of missing some true cases of a disease than to err in the direction of including illnesses that are not actually the disease under study. If too many false cases of Lyme disease are included in the studies, for example, then the research and epidemiology data may be distorted and, as a consequence, predictions about the impact and spread of the disease may be inaccurate. Another rationale for the use of strict case definitions is that it enhances the accuracy of new theories about disease causation and new diagnostic tests, and results in more effective new therapies. If the new theory, laboratory test, or treatment works for cases that are conclusive by strict criteria, then it is likely that it will work for a case of the same disease that falls short of the case definition.

Suppose, for example, that a new antibiotic has been discovered, and that it is shown to be very effective in the laboratory against *B. burgdorferi*. If the clinical trial of the antibiotic includes several people with fibromyalgia or CFS, which would not be expected to respond to an antibiotic, then the antibiotic's effectiveness in treating people with chronic Lyme disease may be underestimated, since some of the people receiving the new antibiotic *for the treatment of Lyme disease* will not have Lyme disease and will therefore not get better after taking the antibiotic.

For most practicing physicians, however, the case criteria serve as guidelines, not as laws or regulations. In the future, as the health care system changes, it's likely that those involved in the diagnostic process will become more accountable. For the time being, physicians are not commonly asked by authorities to provide documentation to demonstrate why they made a particular diagnosis. Diagnoses of CFS, fibromyalgia, and chronic Lyme disease undoubtedly are being made in cases that do not fully meet the strict criteria.

From a patient's point of view, this can be a good thing. After all, if the patient just misses fitting what may be an arbitrary definition, does that mean that the patient does not have the disease? When criteria are loosened there may be a chance for a therapeutic cure, not just reassurance and sympathy. The outcome of such a relaxation of standards depends, of course, on the abilities and experience of the physician. A physician skilled in and knowledgeable about the "art" as well as the science of medicine can often, even with a less-than-complete set of information, identify patients who will respond to therapy. A less skillful physician may also hang a diagnostic label on a patient, and in most cases there is little risk for the physician in doing this. As discussed earlier in this chapter, however, if the diagnosis is wrong, then this less scientific process poorly serves the patient.

Within the overlapping definitions of CFS, fibromyalgia, and post-Lyme-disease syndrome (see table) are several shared symptoms: fatigue, aches and pains of the musculoskeletal system, sleep disturbances, and a perception of diminished mental function. Many people suffer for months or years with this constellation of symptoms, but for them a diagnosis may be difficult to come by. Their symptoms do not meet the diagnostic criteria for any disease in the textbooks or insurance listings, including depression and other psychiatric disorders. Other people—who are perhaps more fortunate in a medical system emphasizing strict criteria rather than what the patient actually experiences—have additional symptoms or other factors that point to one of these disorders.

Features of Post–Lyme Disease Syndrome, Fibromyalgia, and CFS

Feature	Post–Lyme Disease	Fibromyalgia	CFS
Lyme disease in past	yes	maybe	maybe
Fatigue unrelieved by rest	maybe	maybe	yes
Activity less than 50% of normal	maybe	maybe	yes
Unrefreshing sleep	maybe	maybe	maybe
Difficulty concentrating	maybe	maybe	yes
Musculoskeletal pain	maybe	yes	maybe
Headache	maybe	maybe	maybe
Sore throat	no	no	maybe
Painful lymph glands	no	no	maybe

Not surprisingly for a disorder defined by symptoms, the concept of CFS has changed with time. The older case criteria emphasized a fairly abrupt onset of the disorder, and CFS has been called "post-viral fatigue syndrome" to stress the association between CFS and a "flu-like" or "viral-like" illness. But there are some people in whom the identical symptoms have appeared more gradually. In the United Kingdom what is essentially CFS has been called "myalgic encephalomyelitis" to reflect involvement of the muscles *(my-)*, the brain *(encephalo-)*, and the spinal nerves *(-myel-)*, accompanied by pain *(-algic)* and inflammation *(-itis)*. But true inflammation of these tissues has not been demonstrated, and the effects may be more generalized than that restrictive name implies.

The major emphasis for the strict diagnosis of CFS is on profound fatigue that is not relieved by rest, has persisted for at least six months, and has reduced or impaired the patient's average daily activity, limiting it to no more than half of what it had been. Other symptoms that are more suggestive of CFS than the other disorders considered here are sore throat, painful lymph nodes in the neck or under the arms, exacerbation of fatigue by physical exertion, and mild fever. The diagnosis of CFS assumes that other diseases that can produce fatigue, such as HIV infection or thyroid disease, have been excluded by the patient's medical history, a physical examination, or laboratory tests.

Several laboratory test results have been associated with CFS. Some of them indicate that the immune system is overactive in some respects and underactive in others. For instance, CFS patients often have elevated levels of total antibodies at the same time as they have depressed activity of some of the white blood cells that are a first line of defense against infections. These findings of mixed immunologic abnormalities may help to reveal the basic mechanism for CFS and post-infection syndromes, but they are not common enough among CFS cases to be useful for disease confirmation.

The more distinctive aspect of fibromyalgia is pain, both that experienced by the patient as a symptom and that elicited by the physician on physical examination. The pain may seem to the patient to be centered in the joints, but actually the greatest involvement is of the musculoskeletal tissues outside of joints—hence the specification of fibrous tissue (fibro-) as well as painful muscles. Fibromyalgia is one of the "nonarticular rheumatism" conditions; another is bursitis. One of the principal phenomena of fibromyalgia is a heightened perception of pain from a stimulus that would not normally be considered to be painful. In other words, the person with fibromyalgia feels discomfort under conditions that most people would not view as painful.

The musculoskeletal pains of fibromyalgia are usually worst in the morning and are accompanied by stiffness, intensified by changes in the weather, and temporarily relieved by heat. In examining the patient, the physician finds specific and well-localized points of tenderness and pain when pressure is applied. The patient's responses to palpation and the number and location of the tender points are important factors in making the diagnosis.

Like a diagnosis of CFS, a diagnosis of fibromyalgia depends on the exclusion of other conditions that could produce generalized musculoskeletal pain of this sort as well as fatigue and sleep disturbances. The laboratory studies that are performed to rule out other diseases do not confirm a diagnosis of fibromyalgia. To date there are no laboratory tests, singly or in combination, that prove the existence of this condition.

In view of the poorly understood nature of both CFS and fibromyalgia, it is not surprising that there is not yet a medicine that can cure either of these conditions. Nothing is equivalent in effectiveness to the antibiotics used to fight *B. burgdorferi* infection. If what is taken as a case of chronic Lyme disease is actually a case of CFS or fibromyalgia, antibiotics would not be expected to help except by means of their placebo or mild anti-inflammatory effects. The best that a patient with CFS or fibromyalgia can look forward to is slow improvement over a period that may range from months to years, or perhaps some decrease in symptoms with medication and rehabilitative measures. Medications commonly used to treat the symptoms of these conditions are aspirinlike drugs, such as ibuprofen, and antidepressants. Exercise programs with gradual increases in physical activity have also proven helpful for both conditions.

Other Disorders at the "Subjective Extreme"
Sick Building Syndrome and the Gulf War Syndrome

What have been called "sick building syndrome" and the "Gulf War syndrome" are two other conditions that are also at the subjective extreme of the diagnostic spectrum. Moreover, like chronic Lyme disease, their features overlap with the symptom complexes of CFS and fibromyalgia. Sick building syndrome is an occupational disease that generally occurs among those working in tightly sealed multistory office buildings. Affected people usually complain of respiratory symptoms such as sore throat, cough, and frequent colds, but other prominent symptoms are fatigue, headache, and the perception of impaired memory and concentration. Unlike patients with CFS, fibromyalgia, or Lyme disease, patients with sick building syndrome note improvement during weekends at home, and after the ventilation of the building has been corrected.

The diagnosis of Gulf War syndrome is by definition limited to people who were present in the theater of operations of the Persian Gulf War. But there are similarities between cases of this condition and those of many people who are thought to have chronic Lyme disease. The predominant symptoms of Gulf War syndrome include fatigue, inability to concentrate, loss of memory, headache, and muscle and joint pains. Like Lyme disease, the Gulf War syndrome may last for many months, or even for years, after the end of exposure to the precipitating agents.

Sick building syndrome and Gulf War syndrome are said to result from exposure to toxins and other chemicals in the air, and not from an infection. (An alternative but less convincing explanation of the Gulf War syndrome is that it was caused by the immunizations given to troops before the military campaign began.) In any case, the fact that the symptoms of these two disorders that are associated with the environment resemble those of what may be chronic Lyme disease indicates that there may be more than one route to the same type of illness. In other words, a person suffering fatigue, muscle and joint pains, and memory problems may not have an infection at all.

Total allergy syndrome is another environmental disorder that has been proposed as a diagnosis. Patients diagnosed with this condition have had similar symptoms to those considered in this chapter. Controlled studies of patients purported to be hypersensitive to a wide variety of substances commonly found in the environment have not confirmed these hypersensitivities, however. Likewise, there is little evidence to suggest that the diagnosis of chronic candidiasis is useful for most patients with fatigue, joint and muscle aches, and many of the other nonspecific symptoms that have been discussed here.

Depression

Depression may affect as many as 10 to 20 percent of the population at some time in their lives. Even in communities with the highest risk of Lyme disease, no more than 10 percent of the population has been sick with the disorder at any time. In other regions the lifetime incidence of Lyme disease is less than 1 percent; in most places it is less than 0.1 percent. In high-risk areas a person is just as likely to be afflicted with depression as with Lyme disease. In areas of moderate to no risk of Lyme disease, depression is a much more likely diagnosis.

Three of the most common symptoms of depression and other disorders of the mood are fatigue, unrefreshing sleep, and slowness in thinking and mental recall. In this and other respects, depression is as much a medical illness as Lyme disease, CFS, and fibromyalgia are. Many people with chronic Lyme disease, CFS, and fibromyalgia are also depressed. Sometimes it is hard to tell where chronic Lyme disease stops and depression begins; and then an important question is which came first. If the depression preceded the symptoms of CFS, broadly defined chronic Lyme disease, or fibromyalgia, there is a good chance that treatment of the depression will also lift the symptoms that call to mind the latter disorders. In other words, the basic problem is depression, and the patient probably does not have an active *B. burgdorferi* infection. But if the depression followed the onset of one of the other disorders, perhaps because of discouragement and frustration about continuing physical and mental limitations, then treatment of the depression may be of benefit in helping the person cope with the fatigue, pain, and other symptoms, but it will not resolve the root cause of the symptoms.

The curious thing about depression is that it can arise more or less out of the blue—that is, without a known precipitating event—or it can follow a loss, such as a death of a spouse or the loss of a job, or a major illness, such as disabling chronic Lyme disease. The end result is the same, though, and the treatment is much the same: medication, psychotherapy, or a combination of the two. In some cases the patient requires hospitalization. A common feature of depression is a hopelessness and extreme discouragement that finds its ultimate and most devastating expression as a suicide attempt. The severely depressed person is helpless to turn the situation around. When one is in a deep, dark hole, it is hard to even imagine the light that lies beyond, even if for the rest of the world the light is only an inch or two away.

This hopelessness and helplessness leads to the opinion, held by much of the public, that depression represents a "lack of will power" or a "weak character" instead of the chemical and physiological change of the brain and functional alteration of the mind that depression actually is. A common misconception is that people can "snap out of it" if they just put their "mind" to it. Some of the most productive, creative, and inspiring people in history have suffered through periods of depression. They would testify that once in the depths of a depression, "the blues," "melancholia"—whatever name might be applied—only time, medication, intensive psychotherapy, or hospitalization will return the stricken person to greater well-being.

How can the physician or the patient tell whether depression is the real cause of the symptoms of fatigue, poor sleep, and various kinds of pain? In Evelyn's case, her physicians concluded that she was depressed through a process of exclusion. They first checked for other diseases and even treated her extensively for what they thought was the likely source of her problems: Lyme disease. There was the expectation that her symptoms were all attributable to an infection and hence that treatment with antibiotics would cure her. When the antibiotics failed to cure her, the effect was to pull the rug out from under her. Although she may have been depressed from the start, the approach that was taken in her case led her to reject that possibility when it was finally presented to her.

Evelyn's physicians were in essence telling her that her illness was her fault and her responsibility, and thereby they and she missed the chance to explore the contribution of depression, emotional reactions to illness, and possible initiating and exacerbating factors. For instance, Evelyn's recent household move, her responsibilities to her family, and the pressures of her job may in combination have had considerable influence at the start and during the course of her illness. And if Evelyn's concern about having Alzheimer's disease bordered on being obsessive, her needless overattention to what are normal slips of memory and mental performance may have amplified her view of herself as disabled and doomed to slow deterioration. Finally, if Tad had for a long time been silently but guiltily resentful about her illness, Evelyn's responses to his nonverbal cues may have led to increased tension between them, and further withdrawal by Evelyn.

A tip-off for the presence of depression is a degree of discouragement, self-disparagement, lack of hope for the future, or social withdrawal that is out of proportion to the degree of physical disability. This may be hard to judge because it is difficult for another person to appreciate the disabilities of CFS, fibromyalgia, and some cases of chronic Lyme disease, for reasons already mentioned. Moreover, some people with depression have what are sometimes called "biological" symptoms, such as early-morning wakefulness, change in weight, decreased sexual desire, fatigue, reduced ability to concentrate or plan, and chronic pain without a clear source. These symptoms overlap with those of post–Lyme disease syndrome, CFS, and fibromyalgia. When these biological symptoms are combined with feelings of diminished worth, a persistent pessimism, decreased emotional contact with family members and friends, and lack of motivation for activities such as physical therapy, the presence of depression should be considered. But sometimes only the biological symptoms are apparent in a case of depression; the patient may deny feeling blue, down, or despondent.

There are few laboratory tests or other procedural tests for depression. The diagnosis is almost entirely based on the patient's symptoms and the physician's own observations. Depressed persons have many of the immune system abnormalities shown by people with fibromyalgia and CFS. Even where there are differences between these groups in immunity tests, such as a more typical activation of parts of the immune system in CFS, these tests are not widely available and not adequately standardized. The two objective "tests" that can be useful in discriminating pure depression from CFS and fibromyalgia are a structured evaluation of certain aspects of mental performance, known as neuropsychologic testing, and assessment in a sleep laboratory of the patient's nighttime and daytime sleep and sleepiness. For the former the patient performs various tests and tasks administered by a psychologist. For the sleep testing, the patient spends the night and sometimes part of the next day with noninvasive wires (i.e., wires that don't penetrate the skin) attached to the scalp and the skin over certain muscles. Neuropsychologic testing also serves to identify patients with damage to parts of the brain, and sleep testing can also reveal other causes of fatigue, such as *sleep apnea* (frequent but unremembered awakenings associated with altered breathing patterns).

People with depression are usually first seen and treated by primary care or family physicians. Most people with depression are not seen by a psychiatrist, and even fewer are hospitalized. Psychotherapy can be of benefit on its own for milder cases of depression, and these days the "talking cure" is usually provided by a psychologist or psychiatric social worker, and not a psychiatrist (as used to be the case). Medicines are helpful for some people with mild depression and most people with more severe disease. The two major groups of medicines most commonly used now for treatment of depression are *tricyclic antidepressants* and *selective serotonin reuptake inhibitors*. Examples of the former class of drugs are amitriptyline (Elavil) and desipramine. Fluoxetine (Prozac) and sertraline (Zoloft) are two members of the latter group of antidepressants. Representing antidepressant drugs of different classes are buspirone (Buspar) and bupropion (Wellbutrin), which are being prescribed with more frequency. Less commonly, patients are treated with a class of antidepressants called *monoamine oxidase inhibitors* (MAO inhibitors). These drugs are often effective, but at the cost of a heightened sensitivity to certain foods and some other medications.

All these drugs act by increasing the levels of certain brain chemicals in certain regions of the brain. "Tricyclics" and related drugs work on one group of chemicals, and drugs such as Prozac act in somewhat different ways. Both groups of medicines begin to work only after the person has taken them for a month or two; their antidepressant effects take time to appear, and some patience is required. Both groups of drugs also have other uses besides treatment of classic depression. Low doses of tricyclic drugs have been successfully used for treatment of chronic pain, CFS, and fibromyalgia. The serotonin reuptake inhibitors are increasingly being used for treatment of CFS, fibromyalgia, and post–Lyme disease syndrome.

The effectiveness of these medications in these other disorders is further evidence that an artificial distinction between disorders of the "body" and those of the "mind" is not warranted. Depression, CFS, fibromyalgia, and the post-infection syndrome may overlap not only at the level of symptom complexes but also at the level of the mechanism of disease.

Somatization and Hypochondriasis

Lyme disease, CFS, fibromyalgia, and depression are diseases that arise in a child or an adult and then may either persist or disappear, as a result of the person's own responses, treatment, or both. Other disorders, such as a deficiency of an important enzyme in metabolism, may be congenital—the person may be born with the disease. An example of a congenital disease that does not become symptomatic until the person matures past a certain age is muscular dystrophy.

Some psychiatric disorders don't belong in either of these categories. They are not so much a disordered functioning of the physiology and chemistry of an organ—the liver, the lungs, or even the brain—as they are a style of coping with life and adjusting to one's social environment. These disorders reflect the temperament and personality of a person. Some styles of adjusting are maladaptive, in the sense that the person may not be able to fully enjoy family life, love, and work as well as he or she might otherwise. The behavior of people who are affected in this way may be harmful to those who are close to them as well as to themselves: family members, friends, and fellow workers suffer, too. One disorder that can have profound effects on others is what has been called the sociopathic personality. The "sociopath" lacks compassion for others. He or she cannot experience what it must be like to be "in another person's shoes," and consequently acts without regard to others and without guilt. Some say the sociopath lacks a conscience.

Other styles of adjusting tend not to directly harm other people and society, but they still impair the person's ability to feel comfortable with himself or herself. There are several different types of these disorders of personality, many of them fairly common. These disorders may be attractive personality traits taken to an extreme. And where a personality trait stops and a personality disorder begins can be a matter of opinion. A person who is tidy and well-organized, for example, may be very successful in some professions and in his or her home life. But if the person's need to be neat and clean takes up much of the day with ritualized, unnecessary cleaning and washing, then this "compulsive behavior" would have to be considered an impairment or illness. A man who tends to be skeptical and to question others' motives may be well suited for some jobs, such as law enforcement. But if his suspicions become so intense that he repetitively and groundlessly accuses his wife of being unfaithful, then he is seen as engaging in "paranoid thinking."

Some people have discernible personality traits with regard to perceptions of their body. In their more extreme forms they cause the person suffering, and thus they can be considered disorders. Two of these maladaptive adjustments are *somatization disorder* and *hypochondriasis*. In both disorders otherwise trivial bodily sensations or changes are interpreted inaccurately, at least from what can be broadly defined as the "normal" cultural perspective. Somatization takes its name from the Greek word *soma*, for "body." It refers to the tendency to experience what others might call emotions or mental stress as intolerable or barely tolerable physical symptoms.

We all tend to "somatize" at one time or another. Anxiety is not just a mental state; it is also the tremor of the hands, the increased perspiration, and the hyperactive bowels. Embarrassment is the flushing of the cheeks. Anger is the tense muscles and the clenched jaw. Usually, though, we can identify the change in our bodies as a phenomenon associated with a certain emotional state, or a response to a particular situation. People with somatization disorder—the tendency to somatize taken to a disabling degree—seem to have more difficulty than others in determining this about themselves. The "lump in the throat" is felt as a symptom and not as the result of a disappointment or sorrow. Loose stools and stomach cramps are interpreted as a disease of the intestines and not as a manifestation of underlying anxiety.

Characteristically, people with somatization disorder bring their physician a long list of symptoms and concerns. In fact, somatization disorder is diagnosed if the length of the list and the number of different organ systems involved exceed certain threshold values (and if, of course, there appears to be no medical explanation for the symptoms). Somatizing behavior usually dates back to adolescence or young adulthood. The medical chart may be bulging with work-ups, most of which have not revealed disease of an organ. The diagnoses are of "functional" or "psychosomatic" illnesses, meaning that a pathologic change was not found. In the absence of a long-established pattern of multiple symptoms and medical evaluations, however, excessive somatization may also be a sign of depression.

Whether a patient's somatization is of long or short duration, Lyme disease may enter the list of possible diagnoses for the "illness." Even strictly defined Lyme disease has a long list of possible symptoms, and it may not be an unreasonable diagnosis for a person who presents with headache, joint pains, fatigue, sore throat, forgetfulness, tender lymph glands, muscle aches, and tingling sensations of the hands and feet. Faced with a patient with this complex array of symptoms, a physician may choose to provide the patient with the encompassing diagnosis that he or she may have been seeking: in this case, chronic Lyme disease. The alternatives are to deal with the patient's problem piecemeal, one or two symptoms at a time, or to determine whether beneath the numerous symptoms is a somatizing style. If somatization disorder is present, there may even be a therapeutic response to a diagnosis of chronic Lyme disease, but such gains are usually short-lived. The patient eventually returns with the same or other symptoms.

On the surface, hypochondriasis might seem to be the same as somatization disorder. Both somatization disorder and hypochondriasis have as their basis a faulty set of perceptions, but the maladaptive thinking of hypochondriasis occurs more commonly at a more conscious level than somatization, of which the patient usually is not aware. The hypochondriacal patient is not so much misperceiving bodily sensations as symptoms, as he or she is interpreting the sensations or trivial changes in the body as evidence of a certain disease. In both situations an encounter between patient and physician can lead to a diagnosis of chronic Lyme disease, but it is more likely that a hypochondriacal person has thought of the diagnosis before the physician has. The hypochondriac may admit that he or she worries excessively about cancer but nevertheless cannot stop thinking about whether a newly discovered blemish on the leg is a sign of that disease. Hypochondriacal persons often respond favorably to reassurance alone—at least until the next unfounded health concern arises.

Like somatization disorder, hypochondriasis as a full-fledged psychiatric diagnosis is a disabling exaggeration of a tendency or trait commonly encountered in the population at large. It would be unusual for a person not to have concerns about his or her health. In today's world we are constantly being informed by the news media and public education programs of diseases and health risks. Newspapers and magazines publish simple questionnaires, the purpose of which is to reveal unsuspected conditions, such as prostate cancer or "adult hyperactivity syndrome," in their readers. But the effect of these lists of questions and point-scoring schemes just as often is needless worry about the "disease of the month."

Medical students studying diseases in their pathology classes demonstrate that hypochondriacal thinking can be within the range of normal behavior. The physician-to-be, who does not have the perspective of the practicing physician, worries that he or she has whatever disease is being studied at the moment: "Is that large mole on my back really a malignant melanoma?" Another student wonders, "Is that twitch in my eye a sign of multiple sclerosis?" Recall that Werner, the Viennese medical student, thought that his symptoms indicated a brain tumor.

Some people with hypochondriasis or somatization disorder benefit from psychotherapy. The "talking cure" may be oriented toward achieving insight into the basis of the problem. In this form, psychotherapy customarily lasts months to years. Shorter-term psychotherapy may have the goal of simply changing the maladaptive behavior, with or without insight. Hypochondriacal patients learn techniques to disrupt habits of excessive worry about their health. Somatizers learn through educational sessions to recognize their "symptoms" as manifestations of their emotions, and not of disease. An alternative method of providing care for the person who "somatizes" is to schedule regularly recurring follow-up appointments. This preventive measure shows the patient that the physician has the patient's interests in mind and also provides a means to address new or recurrent symptoms as they arise. If emerging symptoms are dealt with early, an expensive and fruitless medical work-up and perhaps hospitalization may be avoided.

A Follow-Up on Evelyn

■ After thinking it over for a few days, Evelyn reconsidered and visited a psychiatrist. There did not seem to be anywhere else for her to turn. After listening to her story, asking some questions, and reviewing the case, the psychiatrist said that she agreed that Evelyn was mildly depressed. But she added that this was probably attributable to Evelyn's discouragement over her continuing disability. The psychiatrist thought that Evelyn's primary illness most closely matched CFS. The physician was part of an interdisciplinary clinic that focused on people with chronic fatigue, and Evelyn began to visit members of this treatment team for her treatment. A selective serotonin reuptake inhibitor was prescribed for her, along with a gradually progressive exercise program.

By the end of the next year Evelyn had better stamina and usually woke in the morning feeling refreshed. One of her client's books was on the bestseller list, and another's was about to be published. She and Tad still had their difficulties, but they could talk about them with each other now. Evelyn did not resume her frenzied schedule of the past, and in hindsight she found that she had no regrets about this.

Protecting Yourself
from Lyme Disease

9

- Julia had a pet beagle named Barney who sometimes got out of the yard and went into the nearby woods to chase squirrels. Before Barney was allowed back into the house after one of these adventures, someone in the family would check his fur for ticks, almost always finding a tick or two. Julia wondered whether Barney could get Lyme disease, and Julia's mother asked their veterinarian if anything, short of keeping Barney in the house all the time, could be done to protect the dog from the disease. The veterinarian said that the tick checks were a good idea, but he told the family that there was a dog vaccine against Lyme disease. He did not recommend it routinely, because most dogs do not really need it. But it sounded to him that Barney was at particularly high risk. So Barney got a shot that day and was brought back later in the month for a booster immunization.

- In early June one of Werner's friends complained about never getting out of Vienna on the weekends. "Spring's almost over, and we haven't walked in the forest yet," she said. Werner reluctantly agreed to go for a hike in the Vienna Woods. This time he was going to be prepared, though! They wore light-colored clothing with long pant legs and sleeves, and tucked the bottom of their pants into their hiking socks. They applied one insect repellent to their faces, necks, and hands and sprayed another on their clothes. After they came back home they checked each other all over for ticks on their skin and in their hair.

- Catherine returned to her sister's home on Long Island, New York, for an extended visit over the summer. She took her youngest daughter, who was twelve, with her. Two other members of her family, including her nephew, had had Lyme disease in the last few years while living on Long Island. One evening Catherine's daughter noticed while brushing her hair a small embedded tick at her hairline. She had been in New York City all that day, so she must have picked it up the day before, when they went to the nature preserve by the beach. Catherine's sister, with whom they were staying, got clean tweezers and pulled the tick out. She had seen enough of these to know that it was the kind of tick that carried Lyme disease. They called the family physician the next day and asked him whether the girl should be started on antibiotics. When he said that he did not think it was necessary, Catherine called another physician in town who said that he would prescribe a short course of antibiotics to prevent Lyme disease.

■ Roy had fully recovered by the next spring, and he and his wife were expecting their second child. They lived in an area of Westchester County, New York, not far from the shore, and several other people in the neighborhood had gotten Lyme disease. Roy knew that some neighbors sprayed their yards with a pesticide once or twice a year to kill ticks, but he was concerned about exposing his wife to these chemicals while she was pregnant. He knew of one family that had put up a fence to keep deer out of their large estate, but Roy and his wife didn't own enough land to make that worthwhile. Besides, they didn't want to feel as though they were living in a stockade. Roy decided to call a lawn care and landscaping company in the town. The people there recommended that brush close to the house be cleared back and all the leaves at the lawn's edge be picked up.

Each of these people had had Lyme disease and did not want to get it again. Their family members had seen what it was like, and they didn't want to risk getting the disease, either. So these four patients and their friends and family took measures of one type or another to protect themselves and their pets against the disease. Lyme disease can be stopped at different points in the cycle of transmission. Here are seven options for disease prevention:

1. Don't go to or live in a place with Lyme disease.
2. If you do go to or live in a place with Lyme disease, take care to avoid getting tick bites.

3. Reduce the numbers of ticks in the environment with insecticides.
4. Don't feed wildlife near the house during the summer.
5. Prevent deer from entering onto your property.
6. Treat tick bites with antibiotics to stop the infection before it starts.
7. Use a vaccine to provide pets immunity against the infection.

Some of these measures have proven effective and are generally accepted as safe. Others are more controversial, because the "cost" of preventing Lyme disease is perceived as too high by some people and acceptably low by other people. In other cases the effectiveness of the proposed prevention measure is questioned. A few measures, such as a Lyme disease vaccine for humans, are not even available yet.

Protecting Yourself against Tick Bites

How can an individual lower the chances of getting Lyme disease? This is not as difficult as it is for some other infections, like the common cold. There are some routes of transmission we do not have to be concerned about. People do not acquire an infection with *B. burgdorferi* directly from pets, wild mammals, or birds, or inanimate objects, such as a toothbrush or a drinking glass. One person cannot give the infection to another, except rarely through pregnancy or conceivably through a blood transfusion. A condom will not prevent Lyme disease. Neither will a face mask or a filter for water. Eating less fat, giving up smoking, or exercising regularly will not keep you safe from this infection. Lyme disease is prevented by stopping tick bites.

Personal measures against tick bites are appropriate both for a resident of an area with a lot of Lyme disease or for a visitor to such an area. Prevention of Lyme disease around one's home and community will be considered later. Whatever the level of disease prevention— personal, family, or community—the first step is estimating the risk of disease. Practical sense and experience tell us that prevention works—an ounce of prevention, a stitch in time, and so forth. Insurance actuaries go on to tell us, though, that the higher the risk of disease, the more we must pay to cover the contingencies.

Previous chapters dealt with risk assessment and stressed the way in which the incidence of Lyme disease varies widely by location in North America and Europe. Within a single county in the north-eastern or north-central United States the chances of an infection can differ substantially depending on the exact locale. There may be no risk for a high-rise apartment dweller in a housing project but a ten-year risk of 10 percent for a resident of a ranch-style home in the nearby suburbs. The county park with its swimming pools, tennis courts, and closely manicured lawn may pose little risk, but the nature preserve down the road may harbor a lot of disease-bearing ticks. The sandy, windblown beach may be perfectly safe from ticks, but the trek through the shrubs and the woods back to the parking lot may not.

Local knowledge about Lyme disease is not necessarily accurate, though. A man-in-the-street queried about it may be misleading about the risk of the disease. Residents of Connecticut and Montana were surveyed about what they knew about Lyme disease. Connecticut has a higher frequency of Lyme disease than any other state in the continental United States, and there have been two decades of frequent press and television reports on the disease in Connecticut and surrounding areas. People in the Rocky Mountain region may also have heard about Lyme disease, from national news and magazine articles and television programs, but there is no evidence that people are at risk of *B. burgdorferi* infection within Montana's borders. The survey produced good news and bad. Four out of five of the people surveyed in Connecticut knew that Lyme disease was common in their state, although perhaps 20 percent of people in the state still did not know that the disease was a risk. More surprising, however, was the finding that one in four Montana residents polled thought that Lyme disease was extremely or fairly common in their state. There is enough to be worried about in modern life without needless concern about a disease nonexistent around one's home. For up-to-date information about Lyme disease risk, a good source is the local or state health department (see Resources, below).

Having established that Lyme disease transmission occurs in a place, the forewarned resident or traveler becomes forearmed by first knowing what the disease-carrying ticks look like. The differences between Lyme disease vectors and other types of ticks are described in Chapter 3. A reasonable rule of thumb is that if the tick is very small—not bigger than a poppy or mustard seed—then it is a good bet that it is an immature form of one of the *Ixodes* species that carries Lyme disease, babesiosis, and ehrlichiosis; or of *Amblyomma americanum*, a variety of tick that carries ehrlichiosis and a disease resembling Lyme disease in the southern United States. Field guides in libraries and bookstores are sources of other information for distinguishing one type of tick from another.

Ticks need to get to the skin for their meal; denying them access to skin will prevent Lyme disease. Long-sleeved shirts, buttoned up, and long pants with the bottoms tucked into long socks or sealed with tape, cyclists' straps, or rubber bands will provide this barrier. So will closed-toed shoes. The lighter the color of your clothing, the easier it is to see ticks crawling on the fabric. When entomologists collect ticks in the wild, they often use a white fabric dragged over the ground and low shrubs and bushes. Using a cloth that was black or another dark color would make the entomologists' task very difficult.

A novel approach to restricting tick access is a new invention not yet on the market: garters with adhesive and a physical barrier, which are worn on the arms or legs. Ticks apparently cannot move past the bands to the rest of the body. They remain on the distant parts of limbs, which are easily examined.

Once home or back at the hotel, cabin, or camp, the skin and hair should be checked for ticks. This is most easily and quickly done by another person, but a "tick check" can also be performed alone, with the aid of a fine-tooth comb to locate ticks in the hair. Pets should also be examined, especially around their eyes and ears, a favorite spot for ticks on furry animals. Brushing or combing the pet's fur may reveal loose or attached ticks. Some people use a floor mirror to examine dogs. Unattached ticks can be picked off with the fingers or tweezers.

Removing an Attached Tick

If a tick is already embedded on you, someone else, or your pet, there is no reason for panic. The spirochetes are not likely to move from the tick to the person for the first twenty-four to thirty-six hours of the tick's attachment. It may even be more prudent to wait for the proper tick-removal equipment rather than to attempt to disengage an engorged tick with the fingers or a pocket knife. The best tool for tick extraction is a curved forceps or tweezers. (Special tick pliers and extractors that easily fit in a pocket are sold at outdoor sports and pet stores throughout the country, but they only offer a size advantage over proper tweezers.) The points should be sharp enough to grasp the tick's head parts as close to the skin as possible. Once the points are positioned thus, slow, steady traction is applied in a backwards direction, away from the skin. Care is taken not to twist or jerk the tick. Ticks have barbs around their mouth to maintain attachment in the skin, and they are not likely to let go easily. If force is suddenly applied, the tick's body could be ripped off, leaving the mouth and head parts embedded in the skin. If this happens— and sometimes it does, even with good technique—there is probably little harm in leaving the head part there, as if it was a wood splinter. In a matter of days the head part will be pushed up as new skin is formed and the top layers are shed. Trying to remove the embedded tick parts with a knife or other sharp object could lead to skin scarring or introduce infection.

Some people swear by another technique. They say that they can make a tick withdraw by smearing petroleum jelly (e.g., Vaseline) or nail polish remover on the engorged body sticking out of the skin. The theory is that coating the tick in this way deprives it of oxygen, smothering it until it has to withdraw from the skin to get air. As simple and painless as this approach sounds, it is not recommended by most experts. For one thing, it may take several hours to overnight for the tick to be affected. During this time transmission of the infection might occur. One warning that does need to be heeded is the one against using a match or a cigarette to make the tick back out.

Whatever technique is used, the site of the bite should be washed with soap and warm water or antiseptic solution after the tick is removed. An antibiotic ointment might prevent infection from other bacteria but would likely have little effect on *B. burgdorferi*. The spirochete is not affected by most antibiotics contained in over-the-counter skin and wound ointments. Ticks themselves carry few bacteria, but in entering the skin they may have introduced bacteria living on top of the skin to a deeper, more vulnerable layer.

Should the tick be saved? Little is gained from this in most cases, especially if the tick is clearly recognized as the deer tick, *Ixodes scapularis,* or one of the other known vectors of Lyme disease. The only possible value of opening up an *Ixodes* tick is to tell whether or not it is carrying *B. burgdorferi.* If it is not—and odds for this run from 40 to 99 percent, depending on the location—then there is no risk of infection. But this analysis would be difficult if not impossible for most physicians' offices, health departments, or medical schools to carry out. Spirochete detection in ticks requires specialized expertise and equipment, and only a few research centers in the country are capable of doing it accurately.

A better reason for saving the tick is uncertainty about what type it is. Identification of the tick's genus or species can be helpful for at least two reasons. The first is reassurance. If the tick is not a deer tick (or another type of Lyme disease vector), then worry about Lyme disease is relieved, for the tick does not pose a Lyme disease threat. (It may be a type of tick that carries another sort of infection, such as Rocky Mountain spotted fever or ehrlichiosis, though.) A second instance in which tick identification may be helpful is when Lyme disease has not been known in a particular area. Documentation that *I. scapularis* ticks are actually biting people in the region will heighten awareness of Lyme disease among local physicians. This finding would also alert public health officials to the presence of the vector in their area. For tick identification the extracted or removed tick should be put in 70-percent ethyl alcohol, also known as grain alcohol, denatured alcohol, or ethanol. The state or county health department can provide advice on where to send the tick for identification. A local university or college may have an entomologist on the faculty who could tell what type of tick it is.

The person bitten, or the parent if a child was bitten, should observe the bite site for an expanding area of redness appearing within a few days to two weeks. If this occurs, the person should be seen by a physician as soon as possible. An emergency room visit may not be necessary, if the physician can see the patient the same day or the next day. A small area of redness, perhaps raised, that appears within a day or two of a tick bite is more likely a reaction to the bite itself and not an erythema migrans rash. Some people are more sensitive or allergic to tick bites than others, and in sensitive people the saliva of ticks can itself provoke inflammation. This limited rash will usually recede within a few days. If it continues to enlarge and becomes painful or tender, a physician should be consulted. This may not be Lyme disease; instead, it may be a skin infection due to "strep" or "staph" which needs attention and antibiotics. Another indication for immediate medical attention is a high fever (an oral temperature of more than 38°C or 101°F)—with or without a rash—after a tick bite. If Lyme disease is not spreading through the body, the fever may be due to either Rocky Mountain spotted fever or ehrlichiosis, both serious infections. In Europe and Russia, fever, headache, and confusion or drowsiness after a tick bite may be the viral infection tick-borne encephalitis.

Should Tick Bites Be Treated with Antibiotics?

There is controversy about whether to routinely give an antibiotic to a person who has been bitten by a deer tick. The Lyme Disease Foundation medical advisory committee has recommended such treatment. By contrast, the medical advisers to the American Lyme Disease Foundation have not recommended antibiotic treatment as a *routine* measure for tick bites, even in an area with a high incidence of Lyme disease. In studies in the United States and Europe the risk of getting Lyme disease after being bitten by an *I. scapularis* or *ricinus* tick was found to be only about one or two out of one hundred in places where Lyme disease occurs. In general, the risk of transmission is much higher if the biting tick is a nymph or an adult rather than a larva, and if the tick remains embedded for more than thirty-six hours. Another factor in the decision to treat is whether the bitten person resides in an area where Lyme disease exposure is a daily occurrence. It would be neither practical nor safe for people to be continuously or intermittently on antibiotics because of tick bites. If exposure is ongoing, the short duration of treatment for a bite—as opposed to the longer course for a known infection—may temporarily suppress but not eliminate a true infection that had surreptitiously started earlier. Inadequately treated Lyme disease can be difficult to diagnose, because some of the patients who suffer from it do not generate a high enough level of antibodies for a positive laboratory test.

Another factor in deciding whether to take antibiotics for a tick bite is a history of allergies or sensitivities to antibiotics. In one controlled trial of preventative treatment of deer-tick bites, there was greater risk of illness in the group who received antibiotics than in the group that did not. The illness in the treated group was from antibiotic side-effects, which are usually mild but can be as temporarily disabling as early Lyme disease.

A still-experimental post–tick bite therapy is topical application of antibiotics. There is a good rationale for this approach: Lyme disease bacteria remain in the skin for two or more days before spreading to the other parts of the body. Until the microorganisms spread, there is no need for an antibiotic that is distributed throughout the body. The investigators who are exploring the topical treatment approach have tried it out in mice who were bitten by ticks bearing *B. burgdorferi.* They found that if the antibiotic was applied twice a day for three days the chance of infection was greatly diminished. For this effect the topical antibiotic has to be started within the first two days after a tick bite. The most effective remedy was tetracycline dissolved in the organic solvent DMSO (dimethyl sulfoxide). DMSO facilitates penetration of the skin by the drug dissolved in it. Unfortunately, the medicines in DMSO also sometimes get into the blood as well. The mice who were treated in this way with tetracycline in DMSO had tetracycline in their blood.

In any case, DMSO is not approved in the United States for human use for this type of application, so another vehicle for the antibiotics would be needed. Erythromycin in 70-percent ethanol, an antibiotic preparation routinely used for topical skin treatment for acne, would be acceptable for human use, but its effectiveness for this purpose in people has not yet been evaluated.

Tick Repellents

Minimizing skin exposure with suitably long and sealed-off clothing will reduce tick bites, but parents, camp counselors, and job foremen, among others, know that such measures are not always readily or willingly adhered to. Tick activity is usually at its height during the hotter months of the year. Many people opt to risk a tick bite rather than to be confined in uncomfortable long sleeves and pants. Whatever amount of skin is exposed, another protective measure is the use of repellents. The two principal choices of repellents for ticks on humans are DEET and permethrin.

DEET (rhymes with "beet") is the short name for the chemical diethyltoluamide. DEET is the most widely used insect and tick repellent and is applied to the skin in concentrations of 5 to 100 percent. The repellent's effect lasts between four and twelve hours, depending on the formulation and on evaporation, perspiration, and water exposure. A new formulation, originally produced for the armed services in the United States, has a longer duration of effectiveness. The DEET is contained in microscopic capsules that release the active ingredient slowly over time; the repellent effect lasts about twelve hours. This formulation, sold under the brand name UltraThon by 3M Corporation, contains 32 percent DEET. It repels arthropods as effectively as, if not more effectively than, preparations containing up to 100 percent DEET. The microencapsulated form of DEET is somewhat less sticky, smelly, and damaging to certain plastics and fibers than older formulations.

The effectiveness of lower concentrations of DEET is important because DEET can be toxic. It is poisonous if ingested by mouth. The consequences can be shock, seizures, and coma; some people with massive DEET poisoning have died. Health problems can also result if DEET is absorbed through open cuts or the eyes. DEET can also enter the body's interior directly through the skin. About 20 percent of the dose applied to the skin is absorbed into the blood; the chemical can be found in the urine for days after a skin application. If DEET is applied daily in high concentrations for a period ranging from several days to weeks to months, there may be sleep disturbances, irritability, and impairment of memory and concentration. Even occasional use of repellent preparations with more than 50 percent DEET has resulted in extensive skin rashes and blistering on some people.

There are a few people who are particularly susceptible to DEET poisoning because of a rare genetic defect in their metabolism. The effects of this defect may be inconsequential for the person's health until the metabolic activity of the body is stressed by DEET or another similar chemical. People with this apparent susceptibility to DEET have experienced seizures and coma from just a few skin applications of low concentrations of the chemical. Most of the ten or so reported cases have been in children, but a few adults have also been affected. Some of them used larger amounts than is recommended, but no more than what many other people have used without apparent ill effect.

To minimize the risk of side effects of DEET the following precautions can be taken:

1. Avoid repellents with DEET concentrations of more than 40 percent. (In the state of New York, DEET preparations of more than 30% have been prohibited.)
2. When spraying the repellent do not inhale at the same time, and take care not to get the spray in eyes or on lips.
3. Do not apply repellent to a skin area with an open wound or one that is inflamed and reddened.
4. Use the repellent no more often than recommended by the manufacturer; usually one application will last four to twelve hours.
5. Wash the repellent off with soap and water after coming inside for the day.
6. Do not use DEET under clothing.
7. If you are a woman you should restrict the use of DEET on your skin if you are pregnant or nursing an infant.
8. Do not apply DEET to the hands or near the eyes or mouths of young children.

DEET can also be applied to clothing made out of cotton, wool, or nylon, but it can harm some synthetic fabrics. It can damage plastics and should not be smeared on plastic lenses, goggles, or watch crystals. A better repellent for use on clothing is permethrin, a synthetic chemical related to natural insecticides called pyrethrins that are found in chrysanthemums. Permethrin, unlike DEET, also kills insects as well as ticks. It does this by disturbing the function of their nerves. One brand name of permethrin is Permanone, available as a 0.5-percent aerosol spray. In this formulation it is approved for use on fabrics and other surfaces but not skin. Permethrin binds well to cloth and once there holds fast even with repeated exposures to rain and washing with detergent. The effects on clothing can last for up to six weeks. Permethrin sprayed onto socks, pants, and shirts is very effective in reducing bites of ticks and other arthropods. The risk of bites is lowered further still if permethrin on clothing is used in combination with DEET application on exposed skin. A combination of permethrin and DEET in a soap is available in some countries.

Permethrin is also available as a rinse and cream for the skin, but these formulations are only approved for the treatment of scabies, a skin disease caused by mites, the smallest arachnids. These permethrin formulations are safely used on the skin as a single application for scabies, but the effectiveness of this procedure for repelling ticks from the skin has not been tested. Presumably the repellent would persist on the skin after application. This is especially true for people with a lot of body hair, because of the especially strong interaction between permethrin and hair. There is less experience with permethrin than with DEET with regard to toxicity from skin exposures, but the risk of either skin irritation or nerve damage from permethrin appears to be low. Because of the strong attraction between permethrin and fabrics, little of the chemical moves from clothing to adjacent skin. One caution about permethrin is its listing as a *possible* carcinogen.

Other substances that are popularly used as insect repellents are citronella, a natural plant extract, and Skin So Soft, a cosmetic product that has been found to have a secondary use as a repellent for mosquitoes. These products are not known to provide effective protection against tick bites.

There are a variety of products for preventing or treating tick infestation on pets. Flea and tick collars seem to be a simple answer to the problem of preventing tick bites, but they are more useful for preventing fleas than ticks. Their success is greater for smaller animals than larger ones. These collars should not be used around the necks or directly next to the skin of children or adults. Cases of poisoning have occurred when this was done. Some people put flea and tick collars around their pant legs when they go into areas with ticks, but the usefulness of this strategy is untested.

Sprays containing pyrethrins are used for killing loose and attached ticks, but they also would be expected to remain on the animal's fur for several days, thus providing prevention as well. The pyrethrin-based sprays and powders are safer and more effective than flea and tick sprays and dips containing one or more petroleum-based, synthetic insecticides. Electronic repellents for ticks are not effective. There is no scientific basis for their rationale; they have failed every test.

Protecting the Community against Tick Bites
Areawide Application of Pesticides

It's easy for health experts and advisers to make recommendations for personal protection, because the responsibility for disease prevention is placed on the individual. There is no or little cost to companies, institutions, or public agencies, and little tax money is spent in giving this advice. In areas where few ticks are infected, or when exposure is episodic, personal protection measures such as clothing and repellents can lower risk to an acceptable level. However, in areas where tick infection rates are high and exposure is unavoidable, as is true in many suburban environments in the northeastern United States, personal measures alone are not effective. It is not practical, or even desirable, for residents of these areas to dress as prescribed and to use repellents daily throughout the spring, summer, and fall. A study in Connecticut found that people who took precautions and people who did not had about the same risk of infection.

The alternative to a focus on the individual is a focus on the individual's environment. The goal is the reduction of ticks or tick exposures in the environment for a person, a family, a neighborhood, or a community. Unfortunately, less is known about controlling ticks than about controlling insects such as mosquitoes. Application of a synthetic pesticide directly to a tick-infested area is the most common method of tick control. One application of most pesticides is usually sufficient to kill each stage of tick. If new ticks are introduced to the area by host mammals and birds they will not feed again until after they change to the next stage. DDT, because of its persistence in the environment, has a long duration of action. Widespread application of DDT reduced the risk of tick-borne encephalitis in Russia for more than one year, but this was at the cost of residual DDT in mammals and birds.

In the United States at present, the application of chemicals for the reduction of ticks is primarily carried out by individuals on their own properties. Public and health agency acceptance of pesticide use for tick control has been slow because of public fears and complaints about the use of pesticides. Ironically, many of these health departments have been spraying insecticides for mosquito control on public and private lands for years with little protest.

The specific term for a chemical that kills ticks and mites is *acaricide*. Effective acaricides may also be insecticides. Examples are carbaryl, whose brand name is Sevin, chlorpyrifos (Dursban), and cyfluthrin (Tempo). Carbaryl and chlorpyrifos are available in liquid and granular forms at garden supply stores. Both of these petroleum-based pesticides are inhibitors of cholinesterase, an enzyme that facilitates nerve and muscle function. In this effect these insecticides are similar to malathion and to those organophosphates developed as chemical warfare agents. Granular acaricides are easier to use than liquids and can be spread like a fertilizer over lawns and ornamental ground cover. Cyfluthrin is available only to professionals in pest control.

The acaricides are applied once or twice a year. One effective schedule for the northeastern United States is to treat the lawn, the edge areas bounding the lawn, ornamental areas, and adjoining forest first during the last week in May, to kill emerging nymphs, and then again at the end of September, to kill the adults that come out in October. This schedule provides protection through the next spring.

Lawn and shrub treatments will reduce ticks in the area by up to 95 percent. In southern states annual spraying of lawns with an insecticide is routine for controlling dog and cat fleas around homes.

For all their effectiveness, traditional synthetic acaricides and insecticides do prompt varying degrees of fear among many people. Synthetic insecticides are recognized as being toxins for other types of animals besides arthropods. If humans are exposed to carbaryl, chlorpyrifos, or another cholinesterase inhibitor in sufficient quantities, they will manifest temporary but sometimes serious abnormalities of their nervous system. Prominent symptoms of poisoning are excessive salivation and secretion of tears, small pupils in the eyes, and twitching in the muscles. Many of these chemicals can be absorbed through the skin, so it is not just accidental ingestion that is the problem. Although there are antidotes, it is preferable to avoid poisoning through proper and prudent use of these insecticides.

The risk of acute poisoning is accepted as fact. More controversial is whether there are long-term effects of continuous exposure to these chemicals. Patients who have suffered acute poisoning have in some cases developed irreversible abnormalities of their nerves, leading to decreased sensation in their hands and feet. There is also evidence, still inconclusive at this point, of mild but long-lasting deficiencies in mental performance in some people who have recovered from an overdose of one of these insecticides. Unanswered still are questions about the consequences of extended exposures to lower doses of carbaryl, chlorpyrifos, and other cholinesterase inhibitors. Hundreds of thousands of people have had such exposures. If there are any long-term deleterious effects, they seem to be subtle.

Another issue is the leaching of pesticides into the groundwater. Carbaryl has now been detected in the groundwater of six states. Most people would agree that contamination of drinking water with pesticides is undesirable, whether these chemicals pose a large, moderate, or only minimal risk to health.

Because of these concerns about synthetic pesticides, people are attempting to control arthropods with less inherently toxic chemicals. Certain soaps and salts of fatty acids have been known since the eighteenth century to kill insects. They have been further developed in the last two decades, especially in organic farming applications. The soaps act as drying agents or dessicants, disrupting the outer skeleton of arthropods and making them susceptible to dehydration. One advantage of these soaps is their rapid degradation in the environment; they do not persist for as long as most petroleum-based insecticides. Another attractive feature of the insecticidal soaps is their comparative lack of toxicity for mammals and birds.

Some of these soaps, when sprayed on lawns and adjoining areas in the northeastern United States, have been found to reduce deer tick populations. But these preparations also contained pyrethrins, the natural pesticides in chrysanthemums. Therefore the efficacy of the soaps alone for tick control remains unproven.

Targeted Tick Control

Another approach to the problem of tick control follows Willy Sutton's advice for bank robbers: that is, go where the "money" is. In the case of ticks, this means that acaricides should be applied where ticks are most likely to be found: the skin of mice or deer. Animals in the wild may carry about at any time numerous attached ticks. One commercial product, called Damminix, was designed to deliver the pesticide permethrin to the ticks on mice. This would be achieved through the use of paper tubes containing permethrin-impregnated cotton. The principle is that mice will use the cotton to build nests, thereby providing a steady exposure of ticks to permethrin when mice lay down in the nest. Property owners spread the tubes out on the lawn and forest on their land. The larger the property, the more tubes are needed. The cost per application to a single property can be in the hundreds of dollars.

As appealing as this idea is, it has worked in only one of four experimental studies. On an island off the coast of Massachusetts, distribution of the tubes with permethrin-treated cotton did reduce the numbers of ticks in the area, but in three other studies the application of Damminix did not substantially affect tick populations. These other studies were carried out in Westchester County, on Long Island, and in Connecticut, all large land areas. The failure of Damminix in these communities may be attributable to differences between their ecologies and that of the smaller island. There were a greater variety of alternate hosts for the ticks on the mainland than on the island.

A similar approach for reduction of ticks on wild mice is the bait tube. These tubes contain food to attract mice and are lined with permethrin to kill the ticks on the mice. Such bait tubes reduced ticks on rodents in Colorado but not in Westchester County, or on an island off the coast of Maine. In the New York study other mammals, which are of only minor importance as reservoirs for Lyme disease, ate the bait as often as the mice did. The higher humidity along the northeast coast also reduced the effectiveness of the treated bait tubes in those studies.

Another place where ticks congregate is on the skin of deer. There are no or few alternative hosts for adult ticks in most places. If deer can be enticed to a certain location with food as bait, they can then be sprayed with an acaricide. This tricky form of "dipping" would eliminate mature ticks, thereby limiting tick reproduction and eventually reducing the entire tick population in the area. Before a deer-targeted strategy such as this could be put into practice, though, there are unresolved problems, such as what acaricide to use, how to deliver the acaricide to the deer, and where to put the deer treatment stations in a suburban environment.

If animals can be attracted by bait to a location where they can be doused or brushed with an acaricide, they also might be treated with a medicine or vaccine. The medicine to be tried might be ivermectin, a drug used to prevent heartworm in dogs and to treat a parasitic infection of the eyes of humans. Ticks as well as worms are affected by ivermectin. If mice or deer consumed bait containing it, the ticks feeding on their blood would be killed. The drawbacks of this approach are the expense of the medicine and the matter of controlling the dose of medicine each animal would get, to keep a particularly hungry or greedy mammal from ingesting toxic levels of ivermectin. Because deer are game animals, there are also concerns about the presence of these chemicals in deer meat.

No medicine delivered in this way has yet been tested; a vaccine for deer is still speculation. The vaccine would immunize deer against ticks and, if successful, would offer an alternative to pesticides for reducing tick populations. But is there any reason to think that an anti-tick vaccine would work? The evidence, though meager, is encouraging. Biologists know that if animals are bitten enough times by ticks, some will develop immunity to them, to the extent that the ticks fall off an immune host sooner than they would fall off an animal naïve to ticks. A group of scientists in Australia have taken this natural phenomenon a step further by immunizing cattle against tick intestines. When a tick fed on one of the vaccinated cows, the antibodies in the animal's blood destroyed the tick's intestine, thus killing it. A challenge facing those who would vaccinate deer against *Ixodes* ticks, though, is how to get the deer immunized. Most animal vaccines are given by injection; vaccinating deer in the wild by this route would be a daunting task. A realistic alternative is an orally delivered vaccine, like that for polio and typhoid. An oral vaccine would be included in bait laid down for the deer, or would be painted on a salt lick.

The aforementioned tick control methods—whether already in practice or still being tested—all depend on the application of some sort of pesticide, drug, or vaccine to either the environment or the host and reservoir animals. An alternative control measure is a living predator or parasite of the ticks. Finding such a natural enemy of ticks is not easy, however, because ticks feed only on blood and then but once a year. They are also solitary animals, seldom close to other ticks. (Humans are comparatively awash in infectious threats through breathing, drinking, eating, injuries, crowding together, and a variety of sexual acts.) One candidate for this form of *biocontrol* is a wasp that lays its eggs in ticks. This was introduced to certain islands off the coast of Massachusetts to control dog ticks in the 1930s. The tick is host here and is killed when the wasp eggs hatch inside the tick and the immature insects begin to grow. These tick parasites have been raised by the thousands and conceivably could be released over time to reduce tick populations. There are other species of this type of wasp that have yet to be studied in North America.

Vegetation Management: Fewer Leaves, Fewer Ticks

Traditional tick and insect control measures employ areawide pesticides, which some people choose not to use. More restricted applications of pesticides, such as Damminix and bait tubes, are of limited value for most homeowners. Novel strategies targeted against ticks on animals are still untested and may be years away from wide implementation. What else can individuals, families, and communities do to lower the risk of tick bites around their homes? There is a comparatively noncontroversial method that can be put into effect simply: decreasing the number of places around a home where ticks can exist.

Although people have gotten Lyme disease from ticks on their lawns, there are many fewer ticks per square meter of a lawn than there are in equivalently sized areas with trees, high weeds, or shrubs. Why is this? For one thing, lawns are more exposed to the sun, and consequently drier, than more sheltered areas. Ticks need a certain amount of moisture and cover to survive; and forests, fields with shrubs, ornamental plants, and fallen leaves provide both moisture and cover. Clearing the land around a house and removing leaf litter will make conditions less congenial for ticks. One way to clear the grounds is to burn leaf litter and weeds growing near the house or lawn. A once-a-year burn may be sufficient to substantially reduce the number of ticks around a residence. A downside of this approach is that nontargeted animals, such as turtles and birds that nest on the ground and near houses, may be adversely affected.

Wildlife Control

One alternative to controlling ticks is controlling the abundance of wildlife around the home. Because ticks are dependent on vertebrate hosts for their nutrition, Lyme disease vectors can be reduced by limiting the availability of hosts, namely deer, rodents, and birds. Rodents and perhaps birds also serve as reservoirs for the spirochete. One way to limit the numbers of these animals is to discourage feeding them, intentionally or unintentionally, during the summer. For instance, spilled food and pet food outdoors attract mice and other small mammals.

An island off Maine that was home to Norway rats instead of mice was an ideal place to attempt another type of host control. The Norway rat, a pest of urban areas throughout the world, was an introduced species on the island. The rats are little-loved, and consequently the community gave its approval for rat control measures. Poison put out for the rats was effective in lowering the rat population on the island. However, this triumph came at a price. A resident's pet, a terrier fond of hunting rats, became very sick after eating a poisoned rat carcass. After this incident it was difficult to gain approval from residents for this manner of rat control.

Equally controversial have been proposals to eliminate deer populations in an area. This is best attempted on islands, which, because of their geographic isolation, will not likely see the reintroduction of a herd. An attempt to reduce the population of deer ticks on a Massachusetts island by removing deer was successful after nearly all the deer were gone. Attempts to eliminate deer from mainland communities have met with more resistance. Many people value the presence of deer, for various reasons. Informed of the risk of Lyme disease, they are still unwilling to eliminate deer from their community. An unlikely coalition of animal rights activists and hunting advocates has voiced complaints about the killing or removal of deer. There is also the argument that any deer control effort must involve a wide area. Although a deer's range is limited to an area a few miles in diameter, the removal of deer herds from one habitat would sooner or later be followed by their replacement by herds from neighboring areas.

Less drastic than a deer harvest is the use of fences to restrict the movements of deer. If fences are high enough, they will keep deer off your property. The owner of a large estate in New York tried this, with the predictable result that tick populations on the property declined over time. But if one family or community puts a fence around itself, the neighbors or the adjoining community will have more deer to contend with. One community agreed to put up a fence, but people on the other side of the fence were against it. Moreover, fences on this scale are expensive and difficult to maintain.

Vaccines

When sources of an infectious disease are unavoidable and when treatment is either nonexistent or only partially effective, we look to that cornerstone of preventive medicine: a vaccine. Malaria is an example. This parasite infection can be prevented by measures that interrupt at one step or another the disease's transmission by mosquitoes. But now many malaria vectors are resistant to the insecticides that once kept their numbers low. Malaria has been successfully treated with medicines such as quinine. But the malaria parasites themselves are becoming resistant to the effects of these treatments. As the standbys of prevention and treatment reveal vulnerabilities over time, there is keener interest in developing a vaccine to prevent malaria.

Although malaria's global scope dwarfs that of Lyme disease, there are parallels between the two diseases which are instructive with respect to vaccines. For many years a vaccine for use in humans was generally thought of as a low-priority item for Lyme disease prevention, and in fact, some experts continue to dispute the proposition that a Lyme disease vaccine is needed. Tick bites were viewed as being avoidable by means of a few simple precautions for outdoor activities. Moreover, the disease was seen by most physicians as easily treated with antibiotics. There was, in addition, little apparent incentive for a company to develop and market a vaccine against the disease. A vaccine for the more frequently fatal tick-borne disease Rocky Mountain spotted fever was taken off the market for lack of use. Inasmuch as Lyme disease is rarely fatal, the public's acceptance of side effects or actual illness from a vaccine would be expected to be low. What with the amount of litigation against vaccines for proven killers such as whooping cough and diphtheria, how great would be the "bottom line" for a vaccine against a more benign infection? How tolerant, it was further asked, would people be of untoward reactions to a vaccine against an infection that could easily be avoided to begin with, and that could be treated if acquired?

These are discouraging considerations and doubts. Nevertheless, public and professional demand have grown to the point that efforts to develop a vaccine for humans are now under way on both sides of the Atlantic. One justification is the recognition, over the last decade, that the impact of Lyme disease on the health and quality of life in high-risk areas is considerable. In some communities 10 percent of the population have been infected. There has been only limited success to date in controlling the disease by interrupting transmission to people in these areas. For many suburban residents, exposure to infection is almost impossible to avoid. This is especially true for outdoor workers and residents of communities with many deer and infected ticks around homes. Although many early infections with *B. burgdorferi* come to a physician's attention, further experience has shown that infections occur without the rash of erythema migrans having been noticed. In the rash's absence it is difficult to distinguish Lyme disease from a summer virus infection. In these cases the infection may go untreated during the stage in which treatment is most effective.

People with late infection, like those with the early form of the disease, usually respond to antibiotic therapy, but longer treatments are required. Moreover, some patients with Lyme disease involving the joints or nervous system do not substantially improve even after intravenous antibiotics. The arthritis continues for months to years, or the fatigue and achiness persist long after the antibiotics have been discontinued. Notwithstanding doubts about the accuracy of some diagnoses of chronic Lyme disease, the specter of a large number of persons with unrelieved disabilities has been another factor in the increased interest in a Lyme disease vaccine.

But would a vaccine against Lyme disease even work? One tip-off that a vaccine would be useful is if people become immune to an infection after recovering from the disease. If a person has measles as a child, he or she is protected thereafter against having the disease again. The immune system develops a memory of the measles virus, and if the virus makes its appearance again in the body, the immunity can quickly mount a specific antibody and cellular response to stave off infection. The same is true for typhoid and whooping cough, two bacterial infections. The evidence we have suggests that if someone has Lyme disease that has spread beyond the skin—to the nervous system or the joints, for instance—then that person will be immune to *B. burgdorferi*. Some people have gotten Lyme disease at least twice, but in these cases of reinfection the first infection was treated when it was limited to the skin stage (localized early infection).

Another indication that a vaccine for humans would be successful is if laboratory animals such as mice and hamsters can be protected against the infection by an immunization. An immunization essentially is a controlled infection intended to produce immunity. The infectious agent is kept in check in one of two ways: either it is killed, or its virulence is reduced before it is administered as an immunization. For example, the polio vaccine that is given by injection contains killed virus. The polio vaccine that children take by mouth is a live vaccine with an attenuated virus. The live polio vaccine replicates to a limited extent in the person before it dies out. There is enough of an infection that immunity to future exposures to poliovirus develops.

In a study conducted several years ago, laboratory rodents were vaccinated with killed cells of *B. burgdorferi* administered as two injections a few weeks apart. After the second immunization the animals were given more than enough live spirochetes to produce an infection. All of the animals who had received the killed spirochetes as a vaccine were protected against infection. Control animals had been given only plain saline water (for control purposes, they received the identical batch of saline water used to prepare the vaccination). All of the control animals became infected. These findings were the basis for the commercially developed Lyme disease vaccine for dogs, which is on the market and is described below.

A vaccine composed of whole cells would probably not be approved for use by humans. Whole-cell vaccines may have unacceptable side effects, such as a fever or a swollen arm. Rightly or wrongly, problems that may be tolerated for an animal vaccine are unacceptable for a human vaccine. If a dog or cat dies or has a severe reaction to an immunization, the manufacturer is not likely to be sued for millions of dollars. When the Food and Drug Administration approves a vaccine for humans, this approval means that the vaccine has been tested not only for safety but also for effectiveness. The vaccine for dogs was provisionally approved for use by the United States Department of Agriculture only with the expectation that it might work and that it appeared to be safe. Before initial marketing the manufacturer only had to show that the vaccine produced an antibody in dogs, and that a small group of dogs given the vaccine did not become noticeably sick.

The ideal vaccine for humans is a single, purified substance with few if any contaminating materials to distract the immune system or produce toxicity and side effects. The vaccine currently given for tetanus comes close to this ideal. The tetanus toxin was isolated and altered in such a way that an immunization results in protective antibodies but not in damage to the person. A more recently developed single-component vaccine is that against hepatitis B, a globally important viral disease of the liver. The hepatitis B vaccine was produced through recombinant DNA, or gene-splicing, technology. One advantage of the recombinant DNA approach is that only one of the proteins of the infectious agent need be produced at a time. This makes purification of the vaccine much easier.

There is hope for a single-component vaccine for protection against Lyme disease. One of the abundant proteins of *B. burgdorferi* has been found, when given as a vaccine, to protect mice and other animals not only against spirochetes delivered by a needle injection but also against those delivered by tick bites. The name of the protein is "OspA," for Outer Surface Protein A. This protein is located at the spirochete's surface. The gene—the DNA blueprint—for making OspA has been cloned into another bacterium, and consequently, OspA can now be produced in large quantities free of other spirochete products. If *B. burgdorferi* does provoke an autoimmune response in some people, the chance that a vaccine would cause such a response would be minimized by using a single protein of the spirochete.

At least two pharmaceutical companies are working on a vaccine for Lyme disease based on OspA. In the first studies of its safety in humans the number of side effects was not significantly higher among volunteers receiving OspA than among those given a placebo injection. The next step in the process of obtaining approval and licensing is a large field trial. The first of these was started in 1994. In that year, ten thousand people in New York, Connecticut, Wisconsin, and other locations received vaccinations with either OspA or a placebo. Neither the volunteers nor the physicians examining them later for evidence of Lyme disease knew who had received the vaccine and who got the placebo. If this trial or other trials show that the vaccine has a beneficial effect, it could be generally available within a few years.

If OspA or another protein is successful in vaccine field trials, the issue of who should be vaccinated will arise. Obviously, one factor will be the vaccine's safety. If side effects to the vaccine are common, the risk of disease would have to be high, perhaps as high as one out of a hundred each year, to justify the use of the vaccine. The risk of disease is highest for those people who work or live in areas where Lyme disease is common. If side effects are infrequent and mild, then candidacy for the vaccine could be broadened to include those with only transient exposures to the infection. An example would be someone such as Catherine and her daughter, who annually visit a Lyme disease area for periods ranging from a few days to several weeks. This application of a Lyme disease vaccine would be similar to the use of the vaccine for tick-borne encephalitis virus in Europe, a vaccine that is taken by people with only relatively brief exposures to ticks with the virus.

Is the Vaccine for Dogs Effective?

The question of which people should be vaccinated is still theoretical, since as yet there is no approved Lyme vaccine for humans. The question with regard to dogs is here and now. The first vaccine on the market is called Borrelia Burgdorferi Bacterin. It is produced by Fort Dodge Laboratories. The vaccine is a culture of *B. burgdorferi* cells that has been concentrated. It would then contain not only spirochetes that have been killed but also some substances from the culture medium, such as a protein in cattle serum. Initially, two doses are given, a few weeks apart. The company recommends yearly booster immunizations thereafter. The vaccine was approved for use by the United States Department of Agriculture, and in its first year more than two million doses were administered.

The experimental studies that were carried out to test the effectiveness of the vaccine for dogs suggest that the vaccine works, but the results were not conclusive. In the manufacturer's own study a small number of dogs were tested, and the investigators knew which dogs got the vaccine and which did not. A larger field study of the vaccine was not randomized, meaning that there may have been a bias governing which dogs got the vaccine and which went unvaccinated.

A vaccine for humans would never have been approved for use on the basis of data from such trials. As the reviewers for a professional group of veterinarians put it, "Reports on the efficacy of the Borrelia Burgdorferi Bacterin are encouraging but not definitive." The vaccine appears to be comparatively safe, but the effects of multiple immunizations are not known.

Julia's pet, Barney, was vaccinated after the veterinarian heard about the dog's level of exposure to the infection. Another veterinarian might have concluded that the vaccine was not warranted even with that level of exposure. Most dogs with *B. burgdorferi* infection are not permanently affected—the lameness usually does not last longer than three weeks or so. Like many humans, most dogs with evidence of a past infection have not shown any symptoms that could be attributed to *B. burgdorferi*. In any case, there certainly is no justification for vaccinating a dog to protect its owners from Lyme disease. People get the infection not directly from dogs but from ticks on the dogs. And the vaccine will not prevent dogs from carrying ticks. (Initial advertisements for the vaccine implied that if the family dog were vaccinated, children and other family members would be protected from Lyme disease, too.)

The advertisements were also misleading in that risk was attributed to such activities as going on walks, taking family picnics, and jogging, regardless of where in the United States these activities were carried out. Most areas in North America have a minimal or nonexistent risk of Lyme disease. Many of the millions of doses of the vaccine that have been given were undoubtedly a waste of money and may have put the dogs at risk of side effects. Overuse of the vaccine does have economic advantages: there are greater profits for the manufacturer, and greater fees for veterinarians.

Vaccinating Field Mice: The Ultimate Control Measure?

Administration of a vaccine to mice, perhaps in bait or other food, is one proposed strategy for Lyme disease control. The aim would be to reduce numbers of infected mice and infected ticks at the same time. The rationale behind this approach is this: Antibodies in the blood of an immunized animal are known to kill the spirochetes in the tick as it feeds on the mouse. The immunized mouse would be protected against infection, and a tick that fed on the mouse might be cured of its *B. burgdorferi* infection. A problem, though, is how to provide the vaccine in nature. It is one thing to give a medicine or vaccine to your pet, but quite another to provide it to wild mice in a forest.

Another potential drawback of a mouse vaccine is that use of such a vaccine might eventually produce strains of *B. burgdorferi* that are resistant to the vaccine. As we've seen, humans are dead ends for the spirochete. If a resistant bacterium occurs in a person, that person may get Lyme disease, but it is very unlikely that the resistant spirochete would be passed on to other animals or people. However, if a mouse has a vaccine-resistant strain of the spirochete, it would likely be picked up by a tick and from there would spread in the wildlife population. If the same or a similar vaccine is being used for people, its effectiveness could be much reduced.

Conclusions

People trying to prevent Lyme disease around their homes face big decisions. So do those who are repeatedly exposed to *B. burgdorferi* in the course of their work and recreation. Weighing in on one side are personal concerns about the effects of insecticides, repellents, and vaccines, as well as aesthetic and moral concerns for the environment. Weighing in on the other side is the perceived risk of getting Lyme disease. Important for this latter assessment is the estimated "cost" of getting infected. Some people in high-risk areas accept getting Lyme disease as the price they must pay to live in otherwise attractive and desirable neighborhoods. They consider Lyme disease to be a nuisance that involves a trip to the physician's office every year or two and a few weeks of antibiotics. Others in the same communities see the disease as a significant danger—certainly more than a nuisance—to their and their family's health and are less willing to accept the risk. What a community does will depend on the proportions of residents holding these different views of the disease.

If a majority of the people in a community can agree on a strategy for tick control, a community-based program is probably best.

(In many places, citizens can expect to receive little help from local and state health departments, however, because these institutions are already financially strapped and have other responsibilities.) In the absence of concerted action by a community, individuals and families will have to make their own decisions about reducing the risk of Lyme disease around their homes. One aid in this are the tick management packages that some landscaping companies are offering. These are usually a mix of acaricide application and vegetation management. This type of mixed program is known as *integrated pest management*. The emphasis could be on one or the other—or, most effectively, on both.

Personal protection measures, such as repellents and appropriate clothing, are likely to be most useful for people who are occasionally exposed to disease-bearing ticks. There are possible risks of chronic use of repellents such as DEET; and head-to-toe covering is not acceptable to many residents and workers in high-risk areas during warm weather. Whether one's exposure is occasional or frequent, however, periodic tick checks of the body are useful. The benefit of antibiotic treatment after tick bites is controversial: the risks of side effects from the antibiotic may be as high as the risk of disease. A topical antibiotic to prevent Lyme disease after a tick bite is desirable, and the risk of side effects from this would be expected to be low.

Vaccines offer hope for people who are at continuous high risk by virtue of their residence, occupation, or both. The apparent benefit of the vaccine for dogs is encouraging, but the form of the vaccine used in dogs would not be approved for use in humans. The preparation is too crude and there are too many concerns about unforeseen side effects. The availability of a vaccine for humans awaits the outcomes of the first trials of the purer, recombinant DNA–based vaccines that are now undergoing clinical trials in volunteers.

Resources:
Where to Go for Help

National Nonprofit and Governmental Organizations in the United States and Canada

American College of Physicians
Independence Mall West
Sixth Street at Race
Philadelphia, PA 19106-1572

phone: (215) 351-2830

Information on Lyme disease

American Lyme Disease Foundation
Mill Pond Offices
292 Route 100
Somers, NY 10589

phone: (914) 277-6970
fax: (914) 277-6974
voice information service:
(800) 876-5963 ([800] 876-LYME)

Information, brochures, and physician referrals

Arthritis Foundation
P.O. Box 19000
Atlanta, GA 30326

voice information service:
(800) 283-7800

Information, numbers of local or state chapters, brochures

Centers for Disease Control
and Prevention
U.S. Department of Health
and Human Services
Atlanta, GA 30333

phone: (404) 639-3311
fax information service: (404) 332-4555

Documents on Lyme disease can be requested for fax delivery. The specific document numbers for Lyme Disease are 351701 (General Information and Pregnancy), 351702 (Symptoms), and 351703 (Treatment/Prevention)

Centers for Disease Control
and Prevention
U.S. Department of Health
and Human Services
Division of Vector-Borne
Infectious Diseases
P.O. Box 2087
Fort Collins, CO 80522

phone: (303) 221-6453

Lyme Disease Association
365 St. David Street South
Fergus, Ontario N1M 2L7

phone: (519) 843-3646

Information, brochures, newsletter

Lyme Disease Foundation
1 Financial Plaza
Hartford, CT 06103-2610

phone: (203) 525-2000
fax: (203) 525-8425
voice information service:
(800) 886-5963 ([800] 886-LYME)

*Information, brochures, physician
referral, merchandise*

State Health Departments

Alabama Department of Public Health
Division of Epidemiology
434 Monroe Street, Room 900
Montgomery, AL 36130-1701

phone: (205) 613-5347

Alaska Department of Health
and Social Services
Alaska Office Building
P.O. Box HO6
Juneau, AK 99811

phone: (907) 561-4406

Arizona Department of Health Services
1740 West Adams Street
Phoenix, AZ 85007

phone: (602) 230-5820

Arkansas Department of
Health—Epidemiology
4815 West Markham Street
Little Rock, AR 72206-3867

phone: (800) 661-2597

California Health Department
2151 Berkeley Way
Berkeley, CA 94704

phone: (510) 540-2566

Colorado Department of Health
Epidemiology Division
4300 Cherry Tree Drive South
Denver, CO 80222-1530

phone: (303) 692-2700

Connecticut State Department of
Health Services
150 Washington Street
Hartford, CT 06106

phone: (203) 566-5058

Delaware Department of Health and
Social Services
Epidemiology Program
P.O. Box 637
Dover, DE 19903

phone: (302) 739-5617

District of Columbia Department of
Health and Human Services
1660 L Street N.W.
Washington, DC 20036

phone: (202) 727-2317

Florida Department of Health
and Rehabilitation Services
Building 1, Room 115
1323 Winewood Boulevard
Tallahassee, FL 32301

phone: (904) 488-2905

Georgia Department of Human
Resources
Epidemiological Section
878 Peachtree Street, Room 210
Atlanta, GA 30309

phone: (404) 657-6448

Hawaii Department of Health
1250 Punchbowl Street
Honolulu, HI 96801

phone: (808) 586-4580

Idaho Division of Health
450 West State Street
Boise, ID 83720

phone: (208) 334-5939

Illinois State Department of Health
Communicable Disease Program
525 West Jefferson Street
Springfield, IL 62761

phone: (217) 782-7165

Indiana State Department of Health
1330 West Michigan Street,
P.O. Box 1964
Indianapolis, IN 46206-1964

phone: (317) 383-6807

Iowa Department of Public Health
Lucas State Office Building
Des Moines, IA 50319

phone: (515) 281-4941

Kansas Department of Health
and Environment
Mills Building, Suite 605
109 Southwest Ninth Street
Topeka, KS 66612-1271

phone: (913) 296-6215

Kentucky Department for Health
Services
275 East Main Street
Frankfort, KY 40621

phone: (502) 564-7243

Louisiana Department of Health
and Hospitals
Office of Public Health
325 Loyola Avenue
New Orleans, LA 70112

phone: (504) 568-5005

Maine Department of Human Services
Bureau of Health
State House Station 11
Augusta, ME 04333

phone: (207) 287-5301

Maryland Department of Health
and Mental Hygiene
201 West Preston Street
Baltimore, MD 21201

phone: (410) 225-6031

Massachusetts Department
of Public Health
150 Tremont Street
Boston, MA 02111

phone: (617) 522-3700

Michigan Department of Public Health
3423 North Logan Street,
P.O. Box 30195
Lansing, MI 48909

phone: (517) 335-8050

Minnesota Department of Health
717 Delaware Street South East
Minneapolis, MN 55440

phone: (612) 623-5363

Mississippi State Health Department
Office of Epidemiology, P.O. Box 1700
Jackson, MS 39215-1700

phone: (601) 960-7725

Missouri Department of Health
Bureau of Communicable Disease
Control
1730 East Elm
Jefferson City, MO 65101

phone: (314) 751-6128

Montana Department of Health
and Environmental Services
Cogswell Building
Helena, MT 59620

phone: (406) 444-3986

Nebraska Department of Health
P.O. Box 95007
Lincoln, NE 68509

phone: (402) 471-0550

Nevada State Health Division
Capitol Complex, Room 201
505 East King Street
Carson City, NV 89710

phone: (702) 687-4800

New Hampshire Department
of Health and Human Services
Division of Public Health Services
6 Hazen Drive
Concord, NH 03301-6527

phone: (603) 271-4477

New Jersey Department of Health
Infectious Disease Program
Trenton, NJ 08625-0369

phone: (609) 588-7500

New Mexico Department of Health
1190 St. Francis Drive
Santa Fe, NM 87502-6110

phone: (505) 827-0006

New York City Department of Health
125 Worth Street
New York, NY 10013

phone: (212) 788-4204

New York State Department of Health
Corning Tower, Room 1495
Albany, NY 12237

phone: (518) 474-4568

North Carolina Department
of Environment, Health, and Natural
Resources
P.O. Box 27687
Raleigh, NC 27611

phone: (919) 733-3419

North Dakota State Department
of Health
600 East Boulevard Avenue
Bismarck, ND 58505-0200

phone: (701) 224-2378

Ohio Department of Health—Vector
Borne Disease Unit
P.O. Box 2568
Columbus, OH 43216-2568

phone: (614) 752-1029

Oklahoma State Department of Health
1000 Northeast Tenth Street
Oklahoma City, OK 73117

phone: (405) 271-4060

Oregon Department of Human
Resources
State Health Division
800 Northeast Oregon No. 21
Portland, OR 97232

phone: (503) 731-4024

Pennsylvania State Department
of Health
Division of Communicable Disease
Epidemiology
P.O. Box 910
Harrisburg, PA 17108

phone: (717) 787-3350

Rhode Island Department of Health
3 Capitol Hill
Providence, RI 02908

phone: (401) 277-2432

South Carolina Department of Health
2600 Bull Street
Columbia, SC 29201

phone: (803) 737-4165

South Dakota State Health Department
Division of Public Health
523 East Capital
Pierre, SD 57501

phone: (605) 773-3561

Tennessee Department of Health
312 Eighth Avenue North
Nashville, TN 37217

phone: (615) 741-7247

Texas Department of Health
1100 West Forty-ninth Street
Austin, TX 78756

phone: (512) 458-7328

Utah Department of Epidemiology
288 North 1460 West
Salt Lake City, UT 84116

phone: (800) 538-6191

Vermont Department of Health
Division
P.O. Box 70
Burlington, VT 05402

phone: (802) 863-7240

Virginia State Health Department
P.O. Box 2448
Richmond, VA 23218

phone: (804) 786-6029

Washington Department of Health
1610 Northeast 150th Street
Seattle, WA 98155

phone: (206) 361-2914

West Virginia State Department
of Health
Bureau of Public Health
1422 Washington Street East
Charleston, WV 25305

phone: (304) 558-5358

Wisconsin Department of Health
and Social Services
Division of Health
1414 East Washington, Room 241
Madison, WI 53703-3044

phone: (608) 267-9003

Wyoming Department of Health
Hathaway Building
Cheyenne, WY 82002

phone: (307) 777-6004

Provincial Health Departments

[Alberta] Provincial Laboratory
of Public Health
3030 Hospital Drive N.W.
Calgary, Alberta T2P 2M7

phone: (403) 270-1200

[Alberta] Provincial Laboratory
of Public Health
University of Alberta
Edmonton, Alberta T6G 2J2

phone: (403) 492-8911

British Columbia Centre
for Disease Control
Vector-Borne Diseases
828 West Tenth Avenue
Vancouver, British Columbia V5Z 1L8

phone: (604) 660-6074

Manitoba Health Services Commission
Cadham Provincial Laboratory
750 William Avenue
Winnipeg, Manitoba R3C 3Y1

[New Brunswick] Department
of Laboratory Medicine
Saint John Regional Hospital
Saint John, New Brunswick E2L 4L2

phone: (506) 648-6501

Newfoundland Public Health
Laboratory
Forest Road
Saint John's, Newfoundland A1B 3T2

phone: (709) 737-6565

[Nova Scotia] Director of Microbiology
Victoria General Hospital
5788 University Avenue
Halifax, Nova Scotia B3H 1V8

phone: (902) 428-4110

[Ontario] Laboratory Services Branch
Ontario Ministry of Health
P.O. Box 9000, Terminal A
Toronto, Ontario M5W 1R5

phone: (416) 235-5941

[Prince Edward Island] Department
of Laboratory Medicine
Provincial Health Laboratory
Queen Elizabeth Hospital
Charlottetown, Prince Edward Island
C1A 8T5

phone: (902) 566-6302

[Quebec] Laboratoire de Santé Publique
du Quebec
20045, chemin Str. Marie ouest
St-Anne-de-Bellevue, Quebec H9X 3R5

phone: (514) 457-2070

[Saskatchewan] Division of
Laboratories
Department of Public Health
Hill Avenue and Legislative Grounds
Regina, Saskatchewan S4S 5W6

phone: (306) 787-3129

Internet Resources

The Centers for Disease Control and Prevention has a home page on the World Wide Web. The Web is accessible for those with direct Internet connections and software such as Netscape or Mosaic or those with indirect connections through on-line services such as America Online, CompuServe, and Prodigy. The CDC home page address is the following: http://www.cdc.gov. Once on the CDC home page, you can find information on Lyme disease and other infections carried by arthropods under the Division of Vector-Borne Infectious Diseases. The specific address, or URL, for information about Lyme disease is http://www.cdc.gov/diseases/diseases.html. Information on chronic fatigue syndrome will be under the heading Viral Diseases.

Two nonprofit institutions have established dedicated home pages dealing with Lyme disease. The home page of the American Lyme Disease Foundation (http://www.w2.com/docs2/d5/lyme.html) has up-to-date information on Lyme disease, including prevention of the disease around the home and during recreational and work activities. The home page of the Lyme Disease Network of New Jersey (http://www.lehigh.edu/lists/lymenet-l), in general, contains information from groups and individuals who think that Lyme disease should be more broadly defined than is recommended by most governmental and academic experts.

LymeNet is an electronic newsletter, distributed from a site at Lehigh University, and an on-line service called the National LymeNet, maintained by the Lyme Disease Network of New Jersey. The newsletter is published about once a month and often contains reports on scientific meetings on Lyme disease. Most of the communications to the newsletter are from lay persons. To subscribe to the LymeNet newsletter on the Internet you should send an e-mail message to the following address: listserv@lehigh.edu. In the body of the message, you should type "subscribe LymeNet-L" (without the quotation marks), followed by your name.

An Internet newsgroup or discussion group is sci.med.diseases.lyme. According to the charter for the newsgroup, it is "intended for discussion about many different aspects of Lyme disease as experienced by patients, their caregivers, friends and family members, doctors, or other medical professionals, or anyone affected by or involved with Lyme disease." The newsgroup is not moderated, which means that queries and comments are not edited or otherwise altered or screened.

Index

Library of Congress
Cataloging-in-Publication Data

Barbour, Alan G., M.D.
    Lyme disease: the cause, the cure, the
controversy/Alan G. Barbour.
        p.   cm.
    Includes index.
    ISBN 0-8018-5224-2 (alk. paper).—
ISBN 0-8018-5245-5 (pbk.: alk. paper)
    1. Lyme disease—Popular works. I. Title.
RC155.5.B37 1996
616.9'2—dc20   95-40308